# Radiographic Neuroanatomy
## A Working Atlas

# Radiographic Neuroanatomy
## A Working Atlas

**Harry W. Fischer, M.D.**

Former Professor of Radiology and
Chairman, Department of Radiology
University of Rochester School of Medicine and Dentistry;
Former Chief of Radiology
Strong Memorial Hospital
Rochester, New York

**Leena Ketonen, M.D., Ph.D.**

Visiting Assistant Professor of Radiology
University of Rochester Medical Center
Strong Memorial Hospital
Rochester, New York

**McGraw-Hill, Inc.**
Health Professions Division

New York   St. Louis   San Francisco   Colorado Springs   Auckland   Bogotá   Caracas
Hamburg   Lisbon   London   Madrid   Mexico   Milan   Montreal   New Delhi   Paris   San Juan
São Paulo   Singapore   Sydney   Tokyo   Toronto

RADIOGRAPHIC NEUROANATOMY: A Working Atlas

1234567890 HALHAL 9876543210

ISBN 0-07-021101-9

This book was set in Optima by York Graphic Services, Inc.; the editors were
William Day and Peter McCurdy; the production supervisor was
Robert R. Laffler; the book and its cover were designed by José Fonfrias.
Arcata Graphics/Halliday was printer and binder.

LIBRARY OF CONGRESS CATALOGING-IN-PUBLICATION DATA

Fischer, Harry W.
Radiographic neuroanatomy: a working atlas/Harry W. Fischer, Leena Ketonen.
p. cm.
ISBN 0-07-021101-9
1. Neuroanatomy—Atlases.   2. Central nervous system—Imaging—Atlases.
I. Ketonen, Leena. II. Title.
[DNLM: 1. Central Nervous System—anatomy & histology—atlases.   2. Central
Nervous System—radiography—atlases. WL 17 F529r]
QM451.F57 1990
611'.8'0222—dc20
DNLM/DLC
for Library of Congress                                    90-13247
                                                              CIP

*To the Scandinavian Radiologists*
*who have contributed greatly*
*to the department at Rochester.     HWF*


*To my three young daughters*
*Irene, Laura, and Emilia,*
*whose encouragement and patience*
*contributed so much to this work.     LK*

# CONTENTS

# PREFACE

The study of the central nervous system is founded on mastery of its anatomy. It is on that foundation that a true understanding of physiology, biochemistry, pharmacology, and pathology can be built. After mastering neuroanatomy through the study of cadaver dissections and cross-sectional demonstrations, students must learn to correlate their knowledge of gross anatomy with its representation by modern imaging technology.

As this atlas is an aid to learning and reviewing normal anatomy, pathologic conditions are not illustrated. To enhance its usefulness as a tool for self-study and self-assessment, the images themselves are not labeled. Our format lets the images speak for themselves without intervening text.

Plain radiographic images of the skull and spine are of course included in the book, but the majority of the images come from angiography and myelography and from computed tomography and magnetic resonance. Nuclear medicine and ultrasound illustrate gross neuroanatomy suboptimally and therefore are not included. Sagittal and frontal plane images afforded by MR are included as well as MR cross-sectional images.

Readers seeking an affordable atlas of general radiographic anatomy should see *Radiographic Anatomy: A Working Atlas* by Harry W. Fischer (McGraw-Hill, 1988).

# ACKNOWLEDGMENTS

Alyce Norder and John J. Allen of Lakeshore Graphic Arts made all the drawings of the neural structures. We are indebted to them for their excellent work and full and prompt cooperation.

Most of the images came from the daily case material of Strong Memorial Hospital and some came from the teaching files of the Department of Radiology of the University of Rochester School of Medicine and Dentistry.

William Smith and Michael Malerk of the medical illustration services of the medical school were most helpful to us in making the photographs. Scott Yohe and Dr. Maury Blumenfeld of the General Electric Company provided the MR angiographic images of the head and neck. Oili Salonen, M.D., Ph.D. (Helsinki, Finland), provided some of the myelograms and arteriograms.

This picture collection could not have been completed without the excellent help of Aileen MacKay and Daniel Prosser and other members of the MRI laboratory and CT staff, to whom we would like to express our thanks.

# INTRODUCTION

In radiography of the living man, identification of the images is based on the path taken by the central x-ray as it passes through the body part. A *posterior-anterior (PA) view* is one in which the x-ray enters from the posterior surface of the body part, passes through the body part, exits from the anterior or front surface, and then reaches the x-ray cassette, which holds intensifying screens and film. The x-rays striking the intensifying screens interact with the crystals of the screen, producing light which exposes the photosensitive film emulsion. The emulsion is then developed chemically to bring out the image. In a PA view, the central ray coming from the x-ray tube is perpendicular to the film and is centered on the center of the part being examined (Fig. 1). An *anterior-posterior (AP) view* is one in which the central x-ray enters from

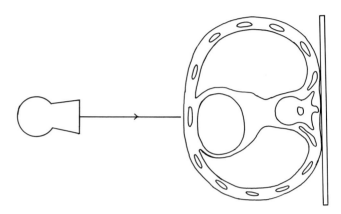
Fig. 2 AP view of the chest.

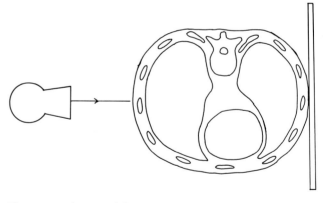
Fig. 3 Lateral view of the chest.

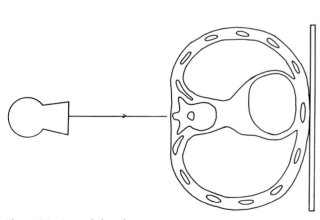
Fig. 1 PA view of the chest.

the anterior surface of the body part, exits from the posterior surface, and then reaches the film (Fig. 2). A *lateral view* is one in which the central ray enters one side of the body part and exits from the opposite side (Fig. 3). These three projections, PA, AP, and lateral, suffice for the majority of x-ray images in clinical practice. In an *oblique view*, the central x-ray passes through the body part at an angle approximately halfway between that of a PA and a lateral view (Fig. 4).

For the skull, a number of different views employ different orientations of the skull in relation to the central ray and the x-ray film. The PA view of the skull, sinuses, or facial bones has the central ray angled 15° to the orbital-meatal line (Fig. 5). The lateral view has the patient's head turned to the side and positioned against the film, while the central ray is directed perpendicular to

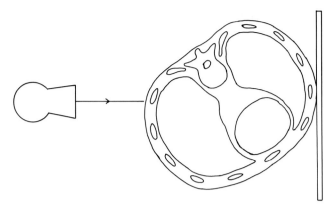

**Fig. 4** Left anterior oblique view of the chest.

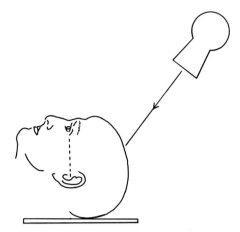

**Fig. 8** Occipital (Towne) view of the skull (see Fig. 5 for key).

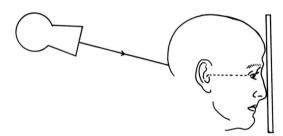

**Fig. 5** PA view of the skull [➤—: represents the central ray; – – – – – – –: represents the orbital-meatal (OM) line, from the angle of the eye to the external meatus of the ear.]

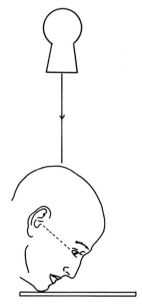

**Fig. 9** PA (Waters) view of the maxillary sinus and facial bones (see Fig. 5 for key).

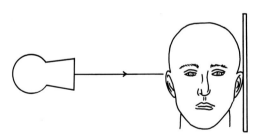

**Fig. 6** Lateral view of the skull.

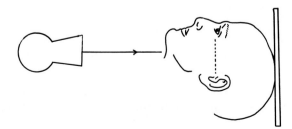

**Fig. 7** Basal view of the skull (see Fig. 5 for key).

the film (Fig. 6). The *basal (submentovertical) view* of the skull and facial bones has the central ray directed perpendicularly to the film and the head tilted back so that the orbital-meatal line is parallel to the film (Fig. 7). The *occipital*, or *Towne*, *view* of the skull and mastoids has the patient supine, with the back of the head against the film and chin tucked down on the chest. The central ray is directed 37° to the feet (Fig. 8). The *Waters view* is a PA view of the maxillary sinuses and facial bones in which the prone patient's chin is against the film, with the nose elevated about 1.5 cm from the film so that the orbital-meatal line makes an angle of 37° with the plane of the film. The central ray is directed perpendicularly to the film (Fig. 9).

For the mastoids there are special views. The *Stenvers view* has the central ray angled 12° to the head of the patient while the prone patient's head is turned 45° to the film (Fig. 10). The *Law view* has the central ray angled 15° to the patients feet and 10 to 15° to the face,

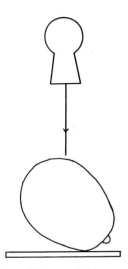

**Fig. 10** Stenvers view of the mastoid.

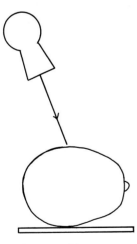

**Fig. 11** Law view of the mastoid.

while the prone patient has the side of the head against the film (Fig. 11).

A view to better visualize the atlas, axis, and the odontoid process of the upper cervical spine is obtained by directing the central ray through the open mouth in the AP projection.

## Imaging Modalities
### Angiography

Angiography in radiology is based on the rapid injection of a volume of water-soluble organic iodide compound (the contrast median) into an artery supplying the circulation of the part to be examined. For the brain and head, injection is made into the carotid and vertebral arteries. Multiple exposures are made as the radiopaque solution flows through the arteries, the capillaries, and the veins.

### Myelography

Myelography, or cisternography, in radiography is based on the injection of water-soluble organic iodide compound into the subarachnoid space by lumbar or cervical (C-1–C-2) puncture. Multiple exposures are made as the fluoroscopic table is tilted, which allows the contrast medium to flow around and define the spinal cord and spinal nerve roots or to fill the cisterns in the head. The water-soluble medium is removed from the body by renal excretion. Air can be used as a contrast medium to define the spinal cord or brain structures, but with the coming of CT and MR, the performance of pneumoencephalography (air cisternography) has practically disappeared from clinical practice. Water-soluble, intravenously administered contrast medium is employed to enhance the vessels in computed tomography. In the normal central nervous system, that is, in those with an intact blood-brain barrier, the contrast medium does not pass from the vessels into the brain or spinal cord tissue. In the remainder of the body the contrast medium passes quickly from the vessels into the extravascular spaces.

The only FDA-approved contrast medium employed thus far in magnetic resonance imaging is gadolinium-DTPA, which is used to enhance lesions. When administered intravenously it does not penetrate into normal brain or spinal cord due to an intact blood-brain barrier. In this feature, gadolinium-DTPA behaves like the water-soluble organic iodides in x-ray angiography and CT enhancement. Gadolinium-DTPA enhancement on MR is not entirely the same as iodinated contrast enhancement on CT. Enhancement of the large blood vessels, falx, tentorium, and dura is not nearly as prominent on contrast MR scan as on contrast CT. However, the cavernous sinus, pituitary stalk, and choroid plexus enhance markedly with contrast. Moderate enhancement is seen in the durea, pituitary gland, and in the small cortical veins.

## CT Images

Computed tomography images are cross-sectional and defined by the thickness of the slice taken, which is usually 1.5, 3.0, 5.0, or 10.0 mm wide. Gaps between the slices are usually not employed. For the skull and its contents the standard planes of the slices are parallel to the supraorbitomeatal line (25° to Reid's anthropologic baseline), and all slices are parallel to each other. The radiologist may select slices of the skull and brain at other angles to the base of the skull. Slices in the anterior-posterior plane or frontal plane are used particularly for visualization of abnormalities of the facial bones, orbits, and the pituitary gland.

## Magnetic Resonance Images

Magnetic resonance, in addition to producing excellent cross-sectional images, also provides sagittal and parasagittal and frontal plane images at the selection of the radiologist. Intervals between slices along with the slice thickness can be varied. The illustrations in the book are picked mainly from daily clinical material. The choice of image plane varies not only because of limitations imposed by patient positioning, but also because special planes are used for ideal demonstration of specific anatomic structures.

## Pulse Sequence

The choice of a pulse sequence requires explanation. One single technique will not display all the anatomy in the optimal way. There are various MR techniques which produce very different appearances of the same structures, depending on the clinical needs.

A pulse sequence consists of one or more pulses of radiowaves. The most commonly used pulse sequence is *spin echo (SE)*, which is defined as a series of alternating 90 degree and 180 degree pulses. The time between the 90 degree pulses is called *repetition time (TR)*.

The intrinsic tissue characteristics, such as proton density, T1- and T2-relaxation times and movement (blood flow) can be displayed in many different ways, depending on the clinical need. For example, the CSF can be demonstrated as high signal (bright) or low signal (dark) intensity on the T2-weighted images. By the choice of TR and TE the SE pulse sequence may be either T1- or T2-weighted. Typically, the SE pulse sequence with short TR and short TE produces T1-weighted images. In these images, CSF, cortical bone and rapidly flowing blood appear as black areas (negligible signal). However, fat (orbit, bone marrow, and subcutaneous areas) appears as bright areas (high signal).

The other commonly used sequences in the clinical setting is long TR with short or long TE. The combination of long TR, short TE (for example 2000/30 msec) produces an image where the signal intensity is related primarily to proton density. In this image CFS has dark signal, fat has bright, and gray and white matter have intermediate intensities. The combination of long TR, long TE (for example 2000/90 msec) produces an image that has a signal intensity related to the T2 values of the tissues. In the T2-weight image, CSF has a bright signal relative to the dark signal from gray and white matter. Cortical bone and rapidly flowing blood have a negligible signal (dark). Fat has a less intense signal than in the proton density image.

Grass imaging (gradient-recalled acquisition in steady state) is a fast scanning technique widely used in spine and head studies.

# Radiographic Neuroanatomy
## A Working Atlas

# PART I

# THE SKULL

# 1/Skull, Paranasal Sinuses, Facial Area, and Orbit □ Skull

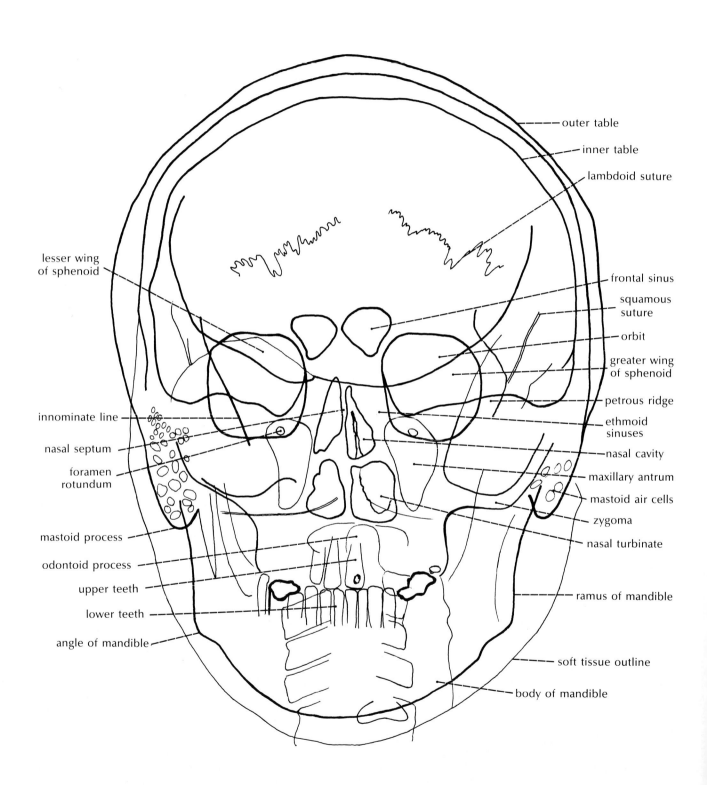

outer table

inner table

lambdoid suture

lesser wing
of sphenoid

frontal sinus

squamous
suture

orbit

greater wing
of sphenoid

petrous ridge

innominate line

ethmoid
sinuses

nasal septum

nasal cavity

foramen
rotundum

maxillary antrum

mastoid air cells

zygoma

mastoid process

nasal turbinate

odontoid process

upper teeth

ramus of mandible

lower teeth

angle of mandible

soft tissue outline

body of mandible

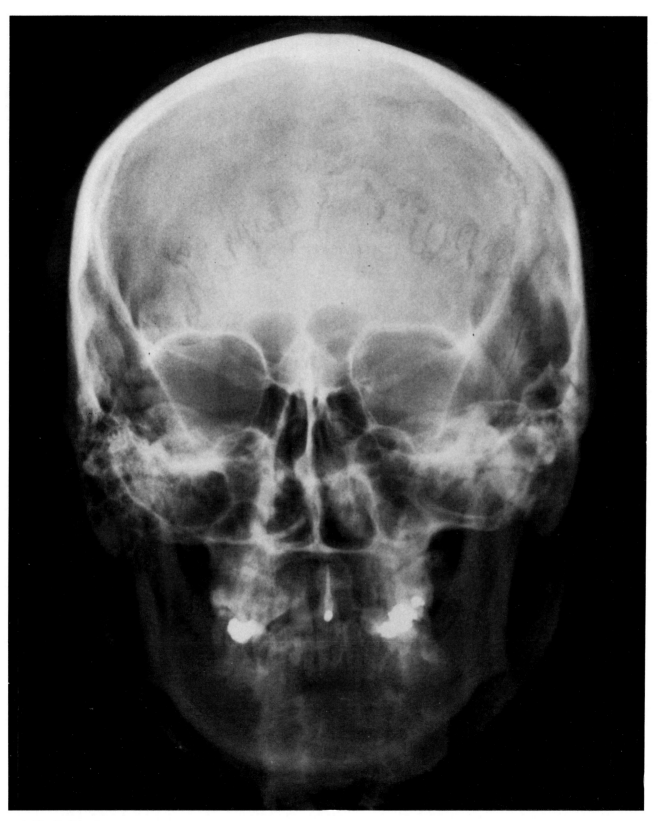

**1-1** Skull, PA view.

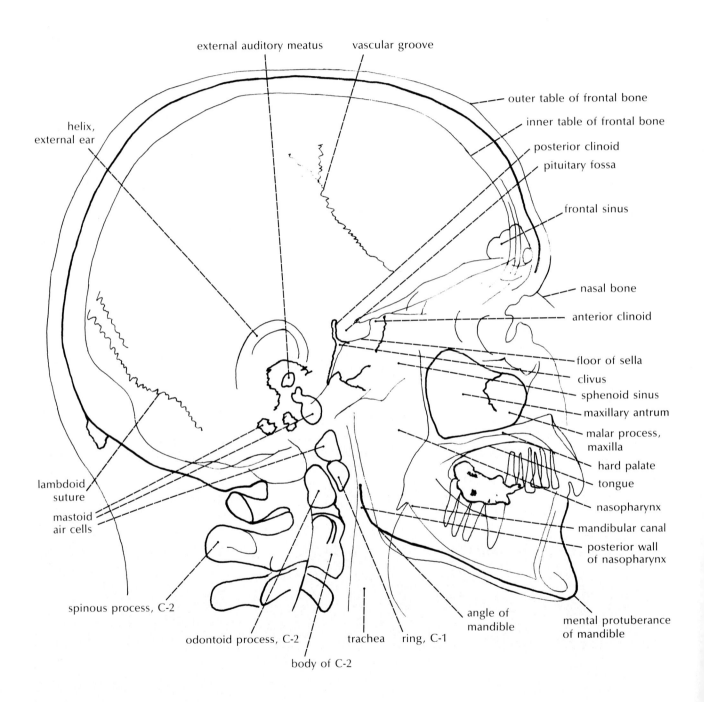

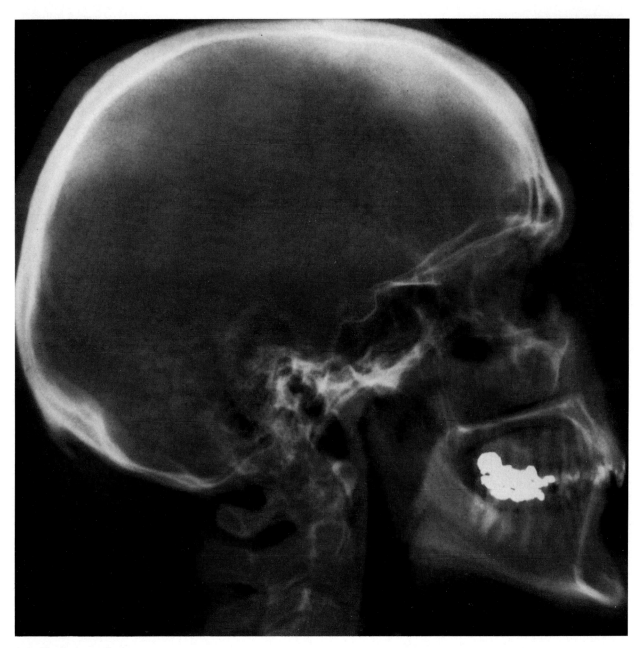

**1-2** Skull, lateral view.

# 1/Skull, X-Ray

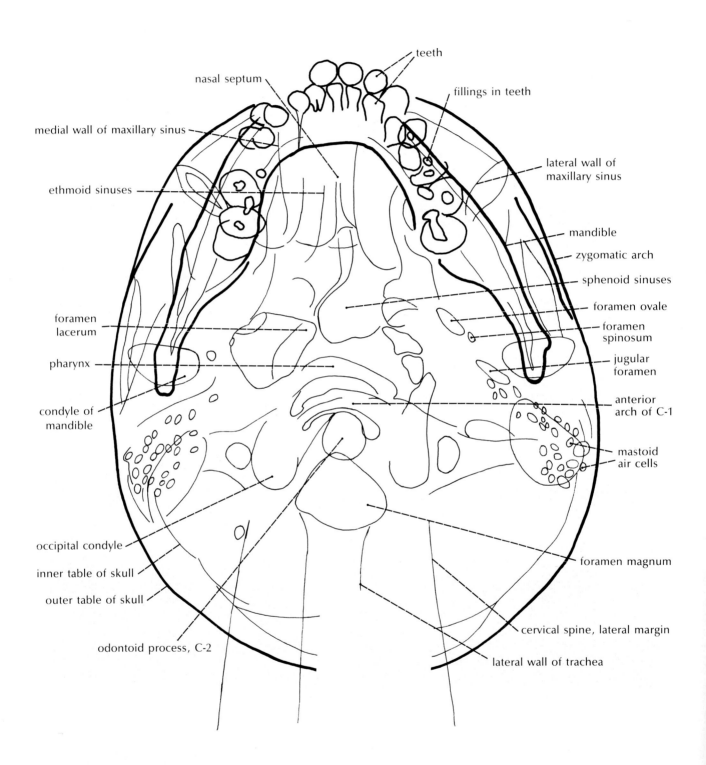

teeth

nasal septum

fillings in teeth

medial wall of maxillary sinus

lateral wall of maxillary sinus

ethmoid sinuses

mandible

zygomatic arch

sphenoid sinuses

foramen ovale

foramen lacerum

foramen spinosum

pharynx

jugular foramen

condyle of mandible

anterior arch of C-1

mastoid air cells

occipital condyle

foramen magnum

inner table of skull

outer table of skull

cervical spine, lateral margin

odontoid process, C-2

lateral wall of trachea

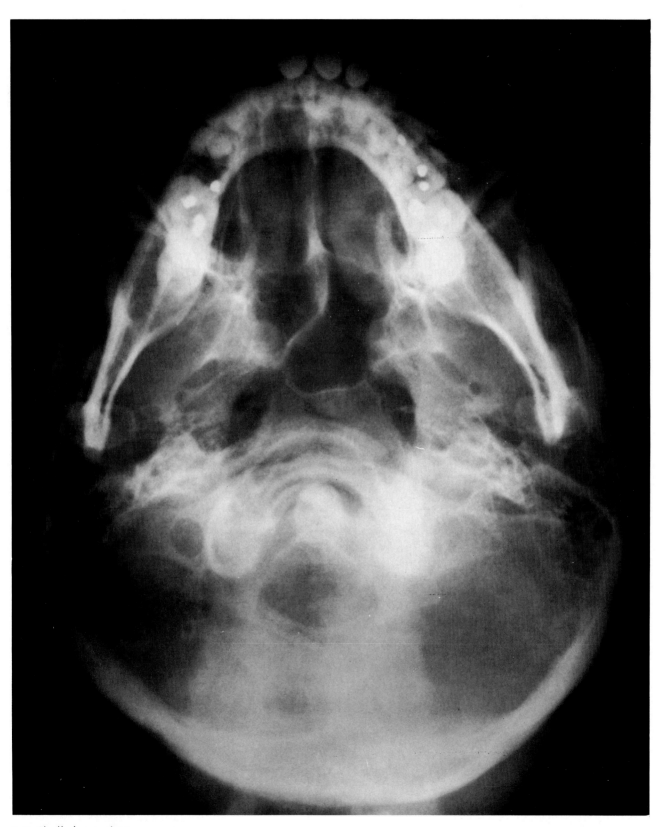

**1-3** Skull, base view.

# 1/Skull, X-Ray

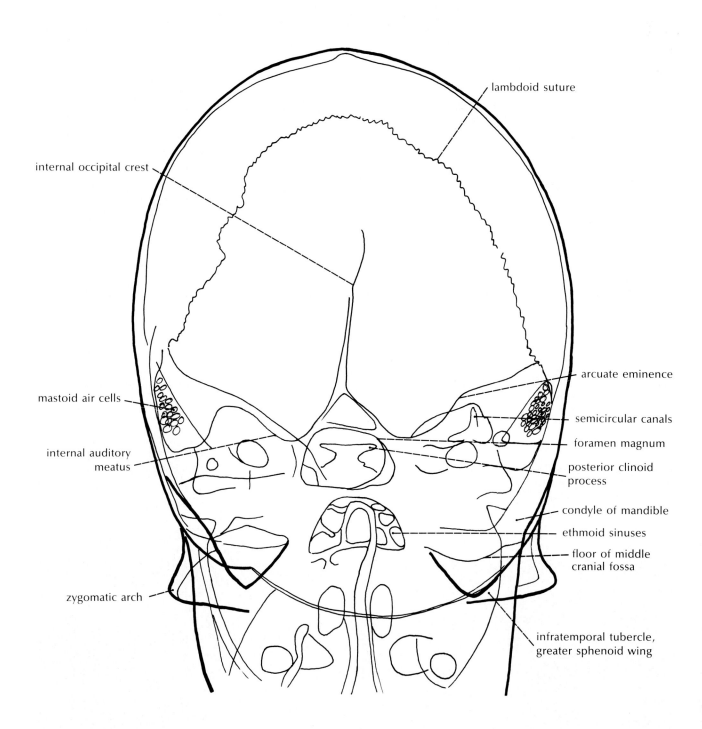

lambdoid suture

internal occipital crest

arcuate eminence

mastoid air cells

semicircular canals

internal auditory
meatus

foramen magnum

posterior clinoid
process

condyle of mandible

ethmoid sinuses

floor of middle
cranial fossa

zygomatic arch

infratemporal tubercle,
greater sphenoid wing

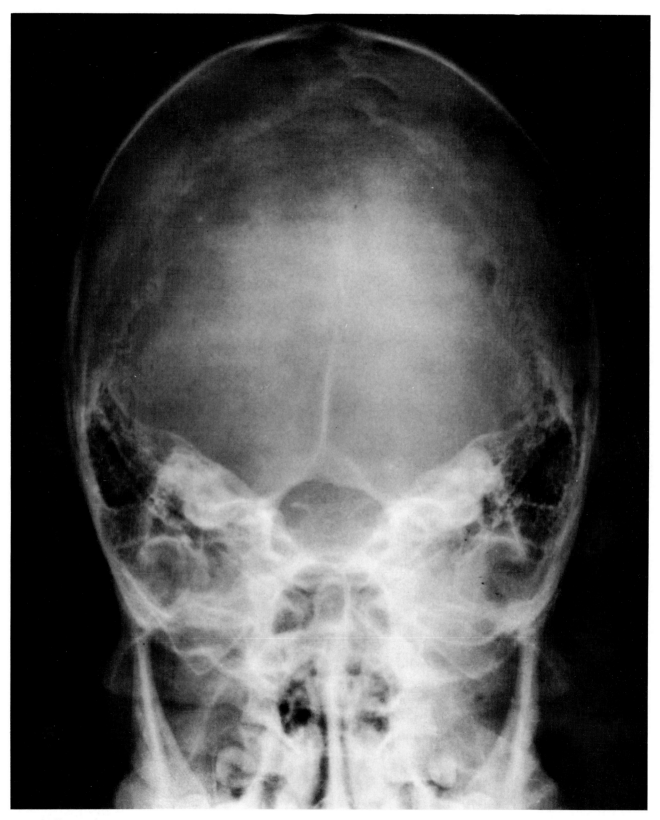

**1-4** Skull, axial (Towne) view.

# 1/Skull, X-Ray

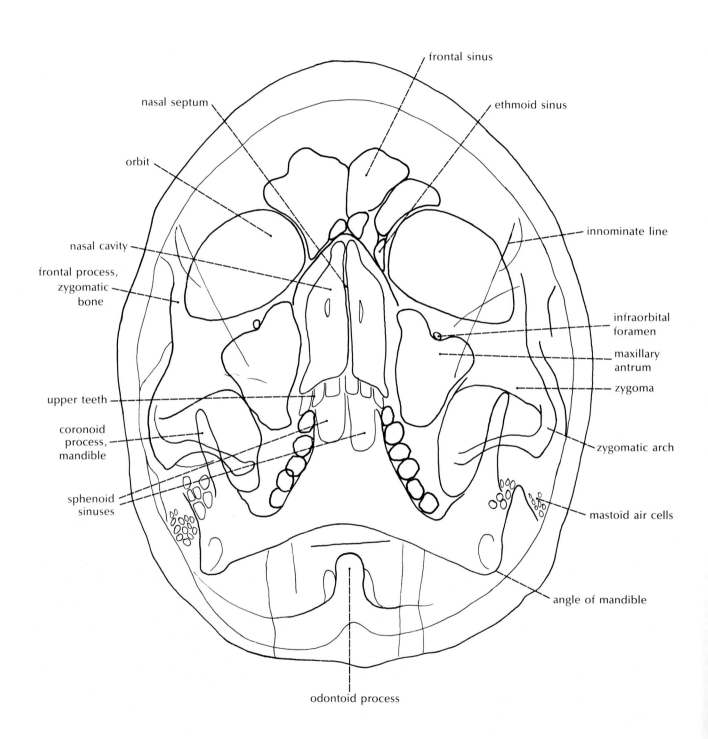

frontal sinus

ethmoid sinus

nasal septum

orbit

innominate line

nasal cavity

frontal process, zygomatic bone

infraorbital foramen

maxillary antrum

zygoma

upper teeth

coronoid process, mandible

zygomatic arch

sphenoid sinuses

mastoid air cells

angle of mandible

odontoid process

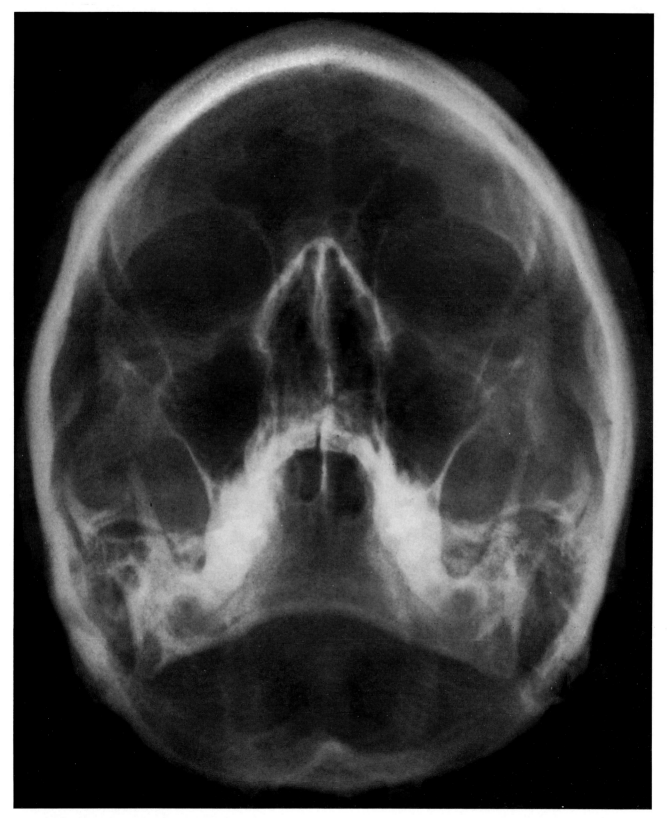

**1-5** Skull, frontal view angled (Waters view).

# 1/Skull Base, Sagittal Scout and Axial CT

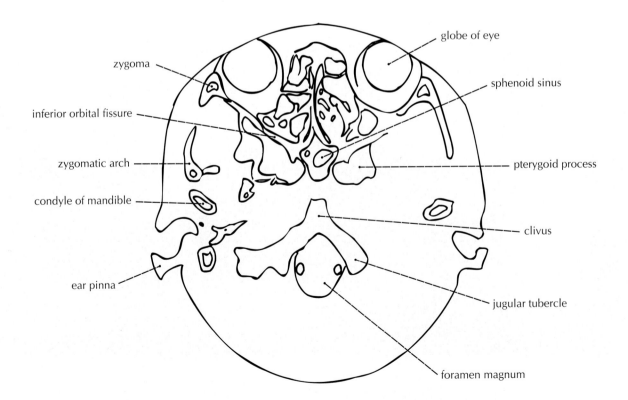

zygoma

globe of eye

inferior orbital fissure

sphenoid sinus

zygomatic arch

pterygoid process

condyle of mandible

clivus

ear pinna

jugular tubercle

foramen magnum

# 1/Skull Base, Sagittal Scout and Axial CT

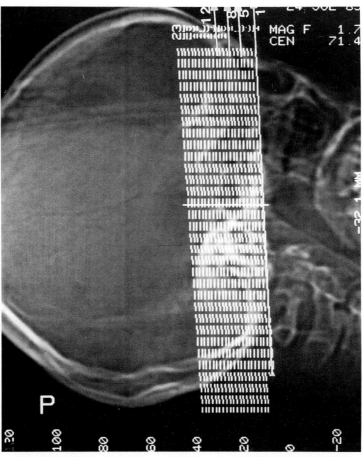

**1-6** A sagittal scout CT scan used for demonstrating the location of selected axial CT scans of the skull base.

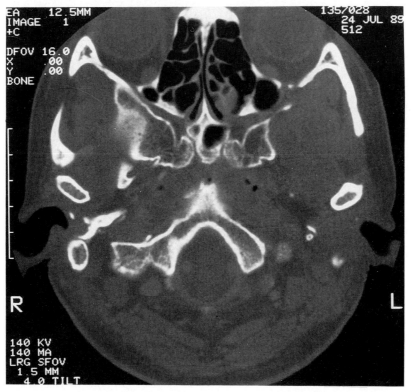

**1-7** Axial CT scan of skull base (section 1 in Fig. 1-6).

# 1/Skull Base, Axial CT

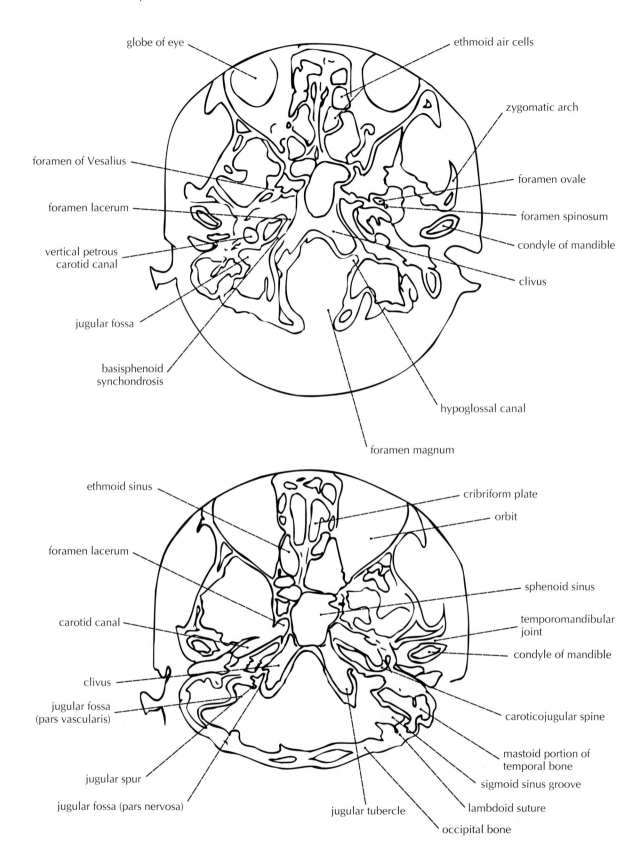

globe of eye

ethmoid air cells

zygomatic arch

foramen of Vesalius

foramen ovale

foramen lacerum

foramen spinosum

condyle of mandible

vertical petrous carotid canal

clivus

jugular fossa

basisphenoid synchondrosis

hypoglossal canal

foramen magnum

ethmoid sinus

cribriform plate

orbit

foramen lacerum

sphenoid sinus

carotid canal

temporomandibular joint

condyle of mandible

clivus

jugular fossa (pars vascularis)

caroticojugular spine

jugular spur

mastoid portion of temporal bone

jugular fossa (pars nervosa)

sigmoid sinus groove

jugular tubercle

lambdoid suture

occipital bone

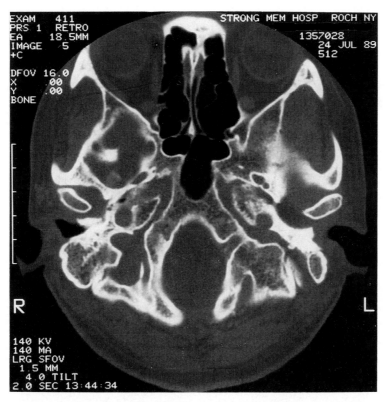

**1-8** Axial CT scan of skull base (section 5 in Fig. 1-6).

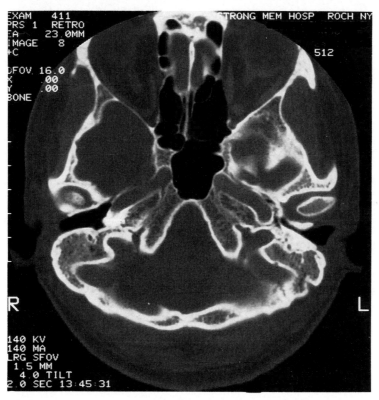

**1-9** Axial CT scan of skull base (section 8 in Fig. 1-6).

# 1/Skull Base, Axial CT

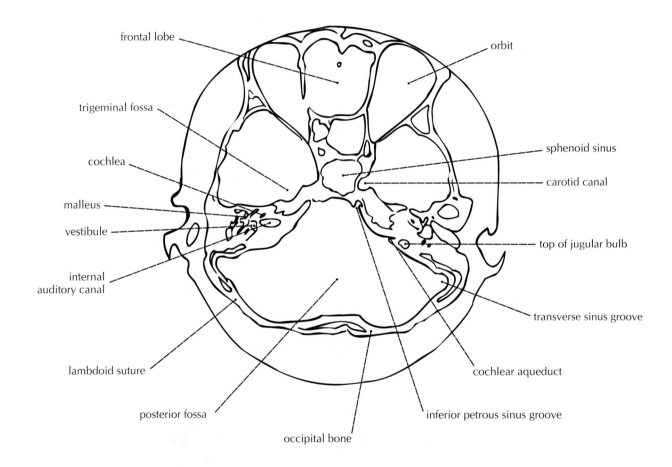

frontal lobe

orbit

trigeminal fossa

sphenoid sinus

cochlea

carotid canal

malleus

vestibule

top of jugular bulb

internal
auditory canal

transverse sinus groove

lambdoid suture

cochlear aqueduct

posterior fossa

inferior petrous sinus groove

occipital bone

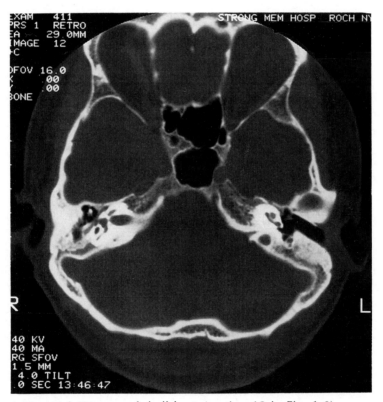

**1-10** Axial CT scan of skull base (section 12 in Fig. 1-6).

# 1/Skull Base, Sagittal Scout and Coronal CT

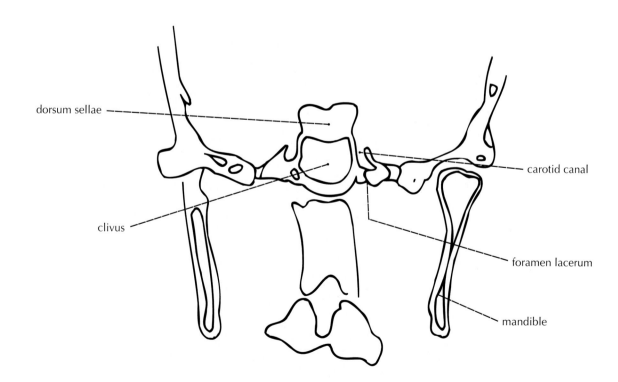

dorsum sellae

carotid canal

clivus

foramen lacerum

mandible

# 1/Skull Base, Sagittal Scout and Coronal CT

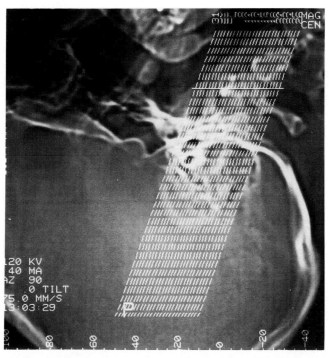

**1-11** A sagittal scout CT scan used for demonstrating the orientation of selected coronal CT scans of the skull base.

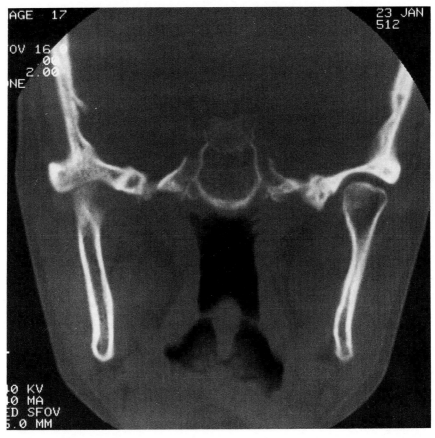

**1-12** Coronal CT scan through skull base. This image is located anterior to section 31 in Fig. 1-11.

# 1/Skull Base, Coronal CT

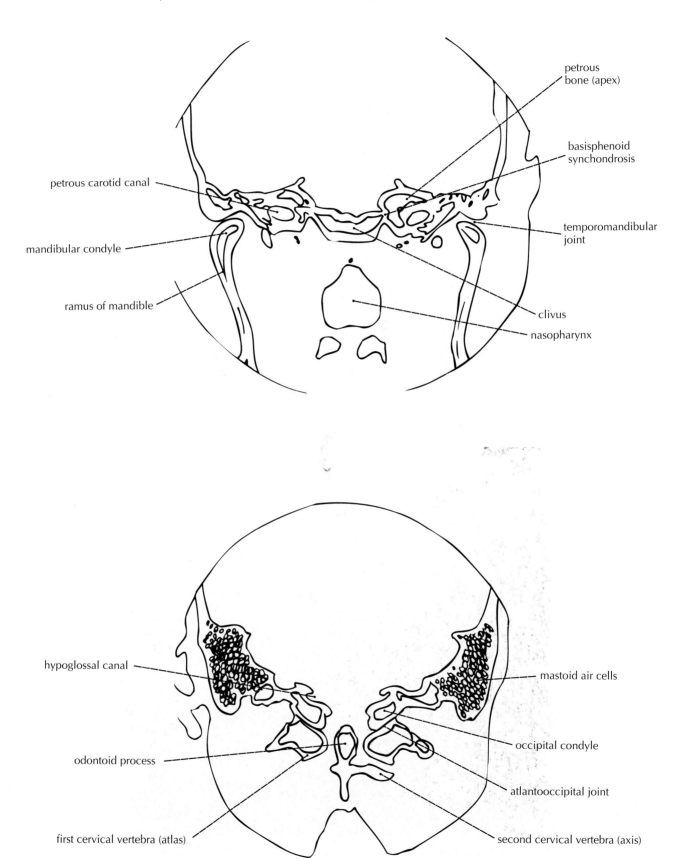

petrous bone (apex)

basisphenoid synchondrosis

petrous carotid canal

temporomandibular joint

mandibular condyle

ramus of mandible

clivus

nasopharynx

hypoglossal canal

mastoid air cells

occipital condyle

odontoid process

atlantooccipital joint

first cervical vertebra (atlas)

second cervical vertebra (axis)

# 1/Skull Base, Coronal CT

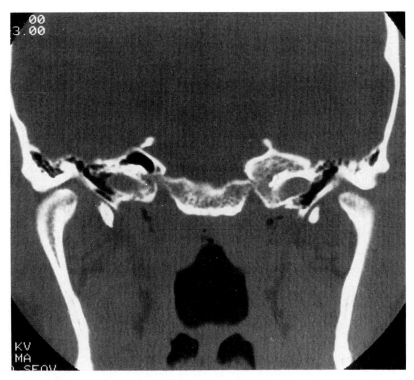

**1-13** Coronal CT scan through skull base (section 30 in Fig. 1-11).

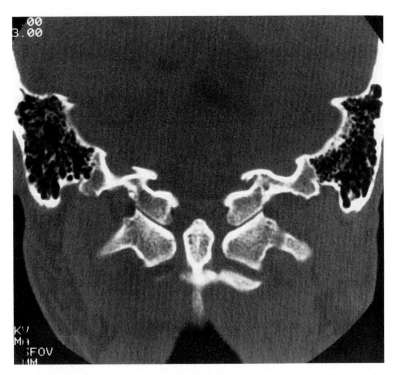

**1-14** Coronal CT scan through skull base (section 17 in Fig. 1-11).

# 1/Skull Base, Coronal CT

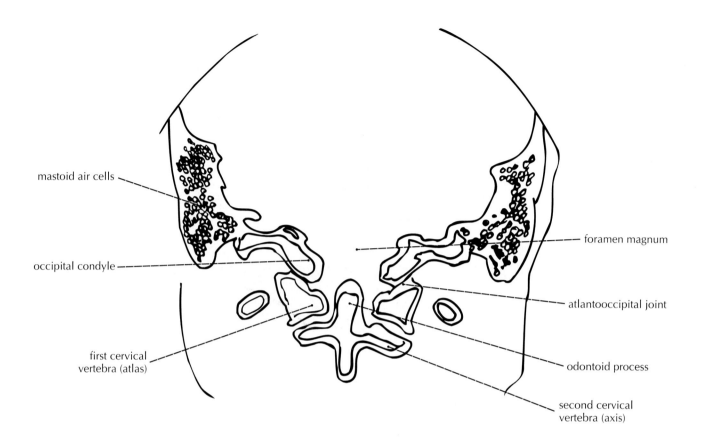

mastoid air cells

occipital condyle

first cervical vertebra (atlas)

foramen magnum

atlantooccipital joint

odontoid process

second cervical vertebra (axis)

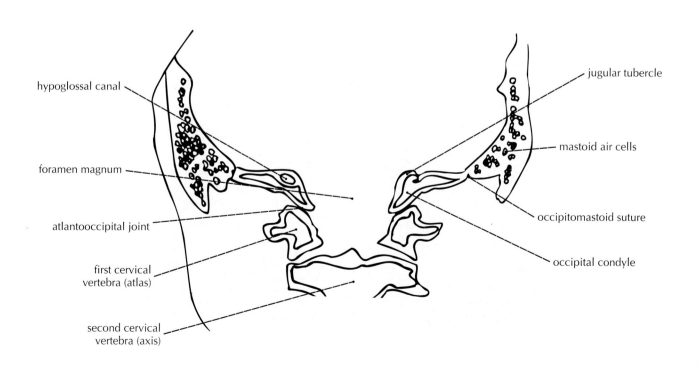

hypoglossal canal

foramen magnum

atlantooccipital joint

first cervical vertebra (atlas)

second cervical vertebra (axis)

jugular tubercle

mastoid air cells

occipitomastoid suture

occipital condyle

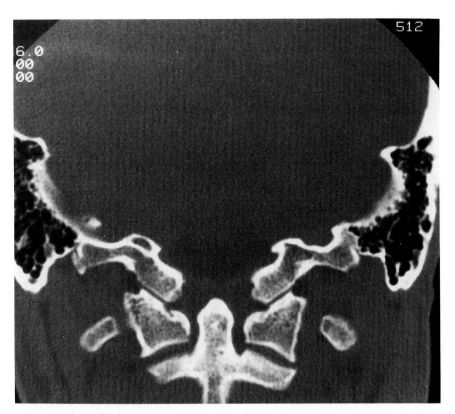

**1-15** Coronal CT scan through skull base (section 19 in Fig. 1-11).

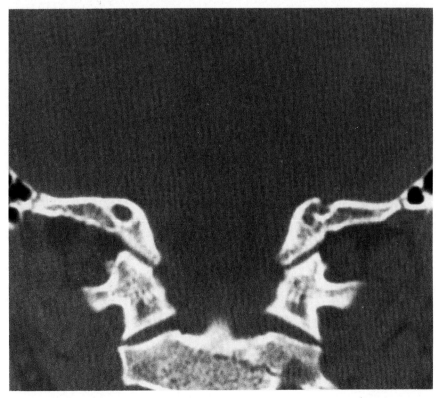

**1-16** Coronal CT scan through skull base at foramen magnum (section 24 in Fig. 1-11).

# 1/Paranasal Sinuses and Facial Area, Scout and Axial CT

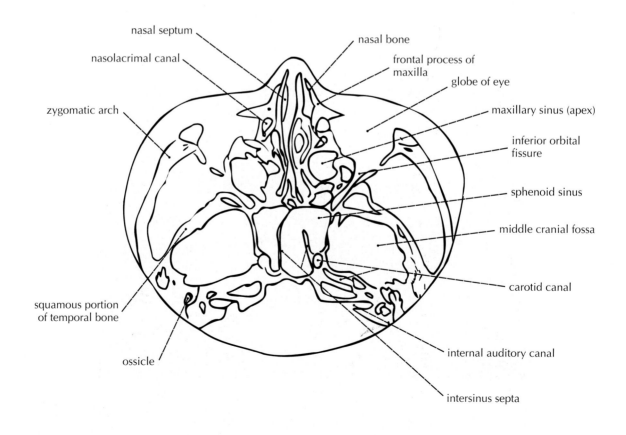

nasal septum

nasolacrimal canal

zygomatic arch

nasal bone

frontal process of maxilla

globe of eye

maxillary sinus (apex)

inferior orbital fissure

sphenoid sinus

middle cranial fossa

carotid canal

squamous portion of temporal bone

ossicle

internal auditory canal

intersinus septa

# 1/Paranasal Sinuses and Facial Area, Scout and Axial CT

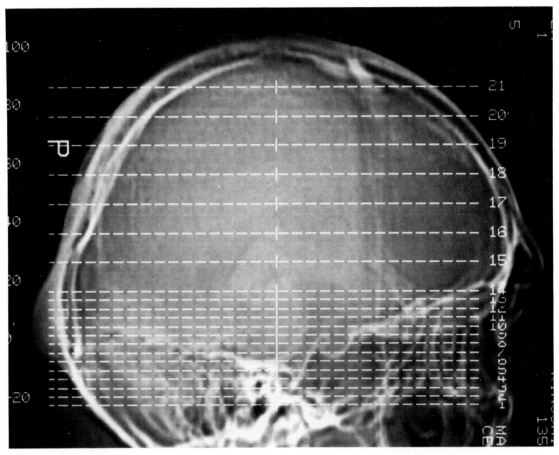

**1-17** Sagittal scout CT scan of the head used to demonstrate the location of selected axial CT scans of the paranasal sinuses and facial area.

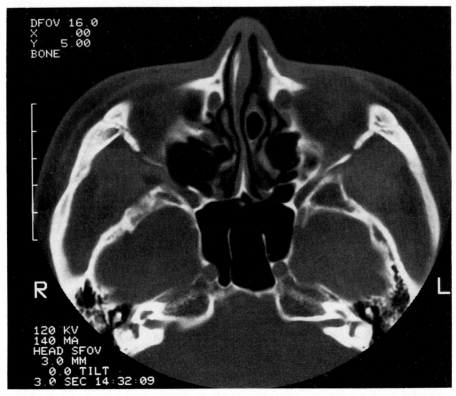

**1-18** Axial facial CT scan (inferior orbit, bone window). Section 3 in Fig. 1-17.

# 1/Paranasal Sinuses and Facial Area, Axial CT

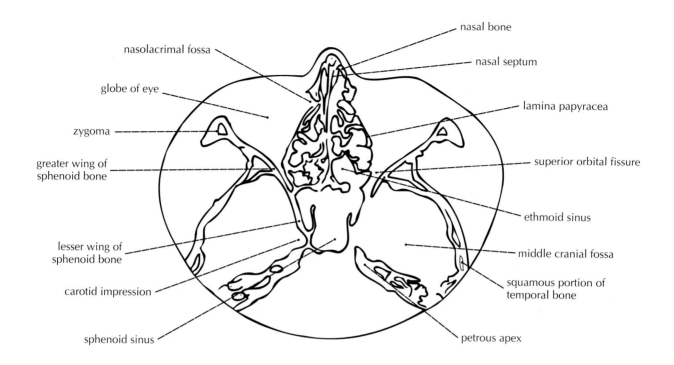

nasolacrimal fossa

globe of eye

zygoma

greater wing of
sphenoid bone

lesser wing of
sphenoid bone

carotid impression

sphenoid sinus

nasal bone

nasal septum

lamina papyracea

superior orbital fissure

ethmoid sinus

middle cranial fossa

squamous portion of
temporal bone

petrous apex

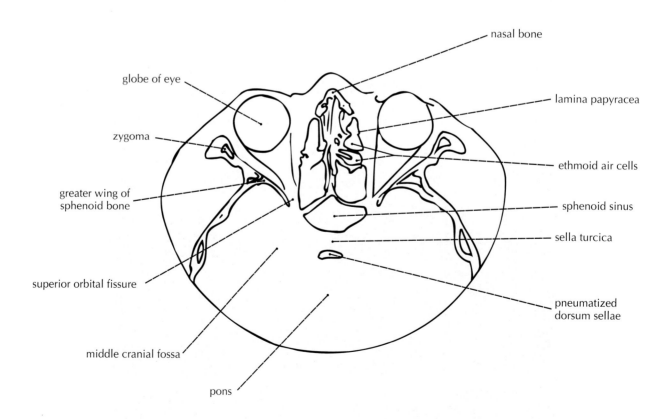

globe of eye

zygoma

greater wing of
sphenoid bone

superior orbital fissure

middle cranial fossa

pons

nasal bone

lamina papyracea

ethmoid air cells

sphenoid sinus

sella turcica

pneumatized
dorsum sellae

# 1/Paranasal Sinuses and Facial Area, Axial CT

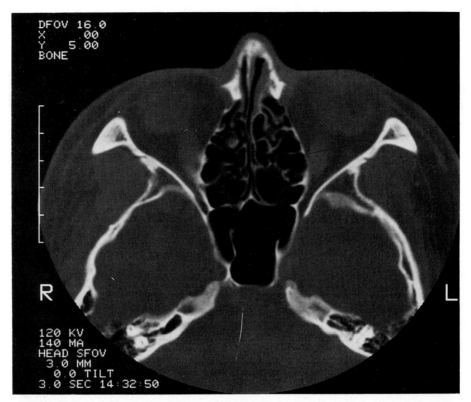

**1-19** Axial facial CT scan (inferior orbit, bone window). Section 5 in Fig. 1-17.

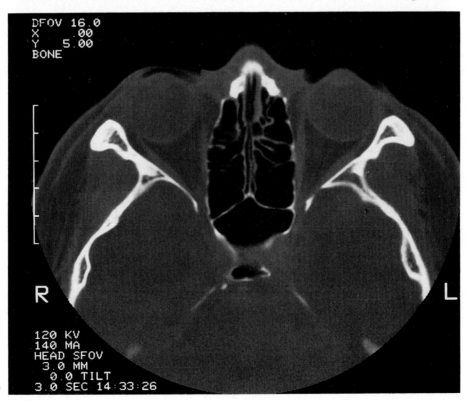

**1-20** Axial facial CT scan (midorbit, bone window). Section 7 in Fig. 1-17.

# 1/Paranasal Sinuses and Facial Area, Axial CT

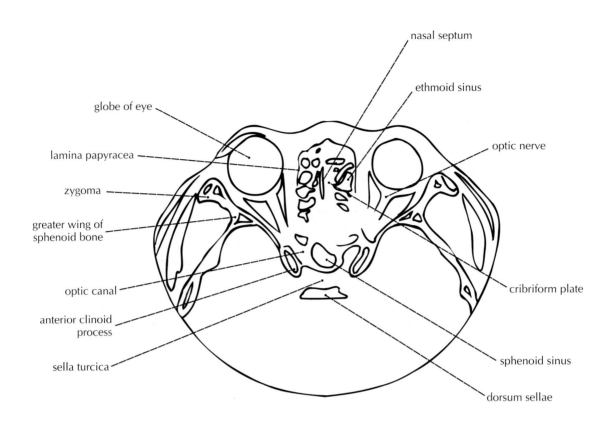

nasal septum

ethmoid sinus

globe of eye

optic nerve

lamina papyracea

zygoma

greater wing of
sphenoid bone

optic canal

cribriform plate

anterior clinoid
process

sella turcica

sphenoid sinus

dorsum sellae

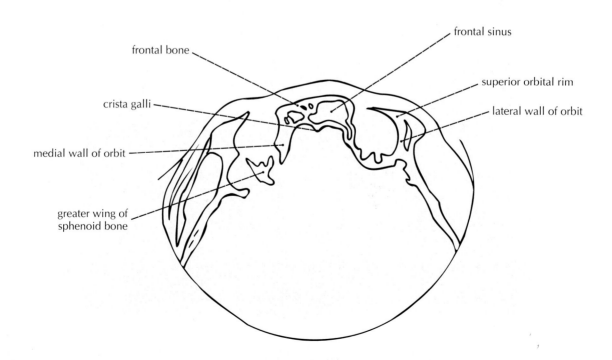

frontal sinus

frontal bone

superior orbital rim

crista galli

lateral wall of orbit

medial wall of orbit

greater wing of
sphenoid bone

# 1/Paranasal Sinuses and Facial Area, Axial CT

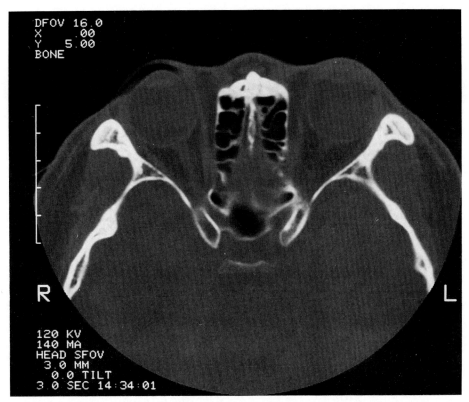

**1-21** Axial facial CT scan (midorbit, bone window). Section 8 in Fig. 1-17.

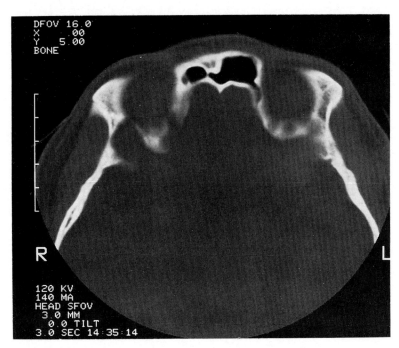

**1-22** Axial facial CT scan (superior orbit, bone window). Section 12 in Fig. 1-17.

# 1/Facial Area, Sagittal Scout and Coronal CT

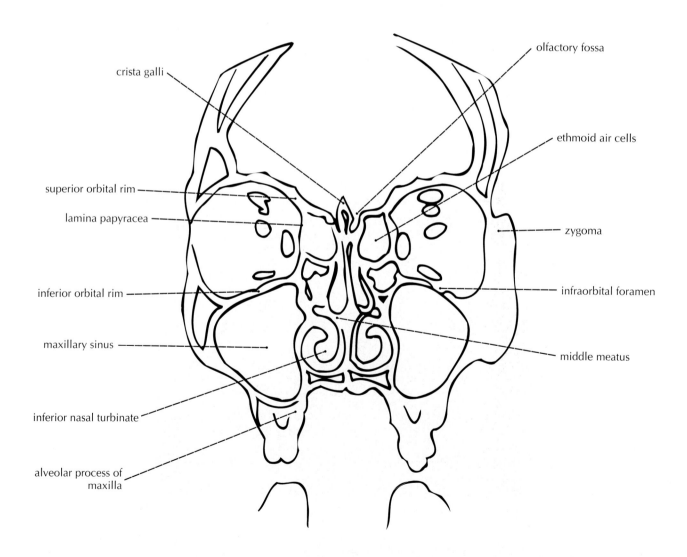

crista galli

olfactory fossa

ethmoid air cells

superior orbital rim

lamina papyracea

zygoma

inferior orbital rim

infraorbital foramen

maxillary sinus

middle meatus

inferior nasal turbinate

alveolar process of
maxilla

# 1/Facial Area, Sagittal Scout and Coronal CT

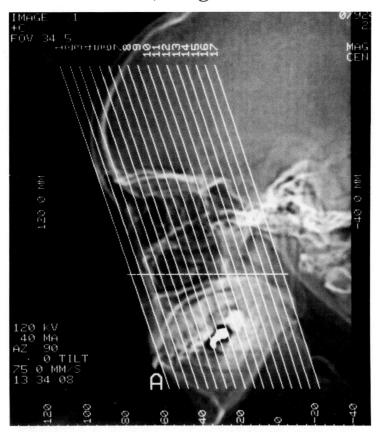

**1-23** Sagittal CT scan used for demonstrating the orientation of selected coronal CT scans of the face and orbits.

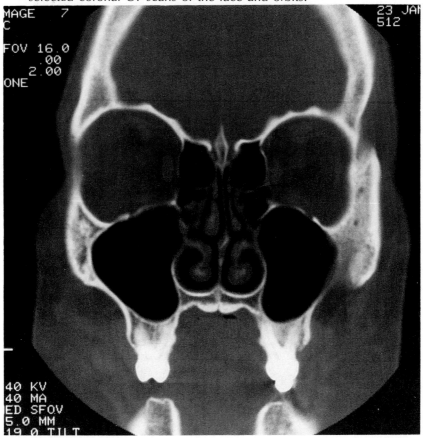

**1-24** Coronal CT scan at level of orbits and central nasal cavity (section 7 in Fig. 1-23).

# 1/Facial Area, Coronal CT and Axial MRI

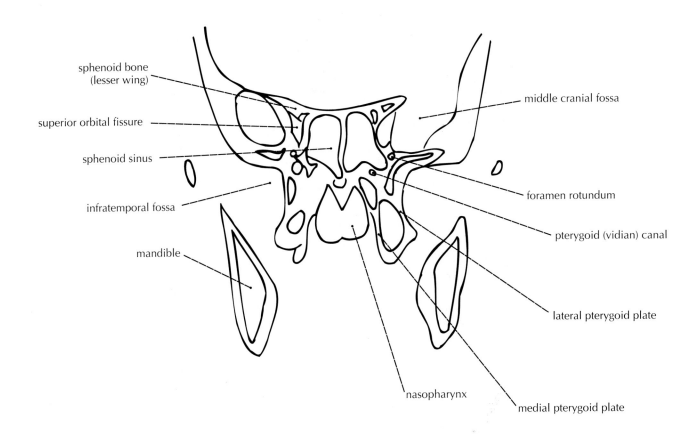

sphenoid bone (lesser wing)

superior orbital fissure

sphenoid sinus

infratemporal fossa

mandible

middle cranial fossa

foramen rotundum

pterygoid (vidian) canal

lateral pterygoid plate

medial pterygoid plate

nasopharynx

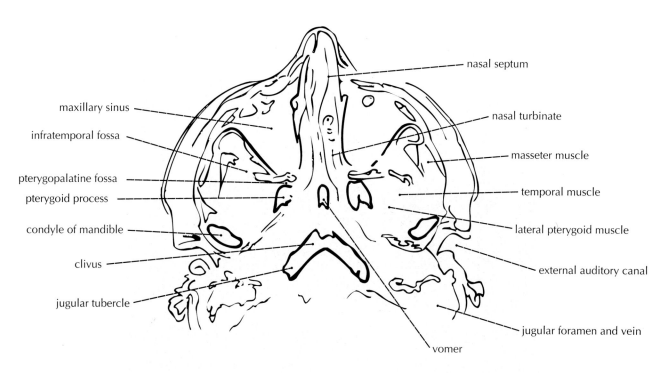

maxillary sinus

infratemporal fossa

pterygopalatine fossa

pterygoid process

condyle of mandible

clivus

jugular tubercle

nasal septum

nasal turbinate

masseter muscle

temporal muscle

lateral pterygoid muscle

external auditory canal

jugular foramen and vein

vomer

# 1/Facial Area, Coronal CT and Axial MRI

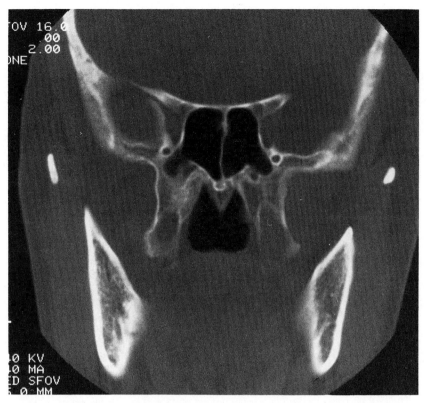

**1-25** Coronal CT scan at level of lesser wing of sphenoid (section 13 in Fig. 1-23).

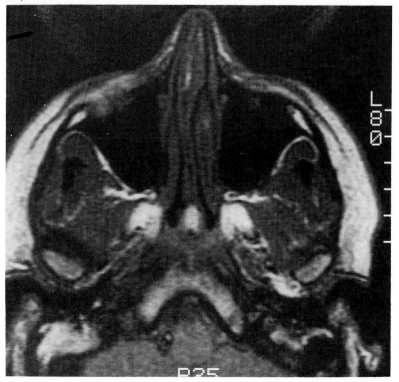

**1-26** Axial MR scan through maxillary sinus and infratemporal fossa (600/20).

# 1/Optic Foramen, X-Ray; Orbit, Axial CT

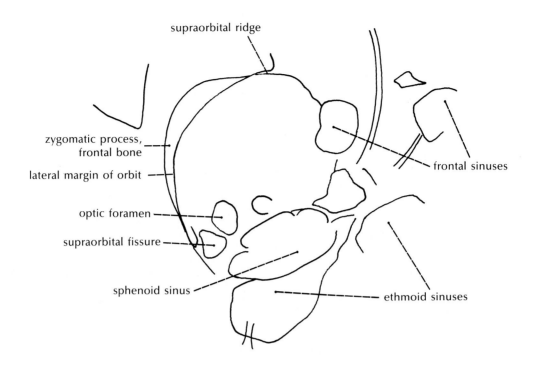

supraorbital ridge

zygomatic process, frontal bone

lateral margin of orbit

optic foramen

supraorbital fissure

sphenoid sinus

frontal sinuses

ethmoid sinuses

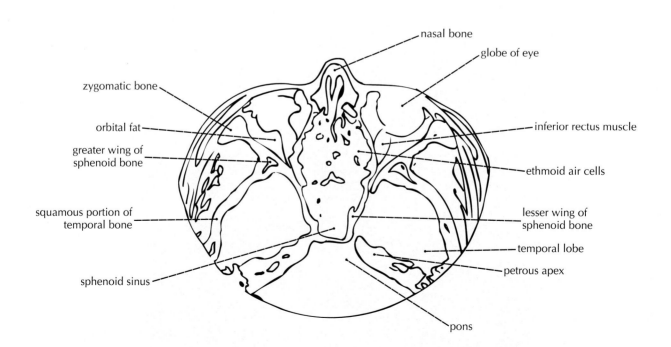

nasal bone

globe of eye

zygomatic bone

orbital fat

greater wing of sphenoid bone

squamous portion of temporal bone

sphenoid sinus

inferior rectus muscle

ethmoid air cells

lesser wing of sphenoid bone

temporal lobe

petrous apex

pons

# 1/Optic Foramen, X-Ray; Orbit, Axial CT

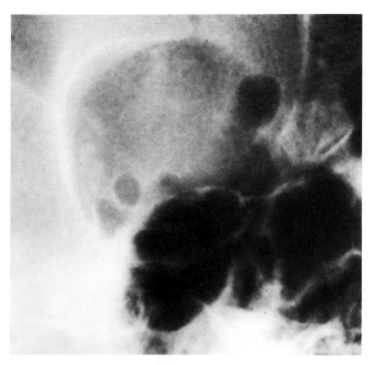

**1-27** Optic foramen, oblique view.

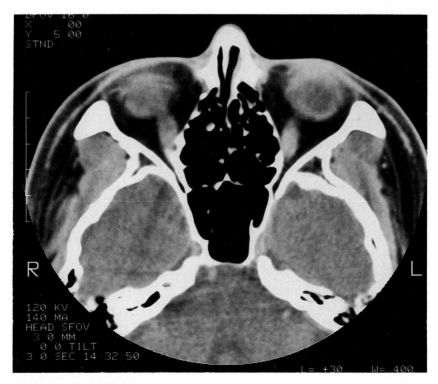

**1-28** Axial orbital CT scan (section 4 in Fig. 1-17).

# 1/Orbit, Axial CT

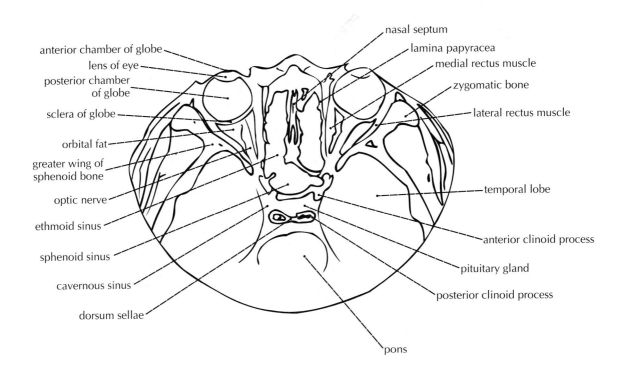

anterior chamber of globe
lens of eye
posterior chamber of globe
sclera of globe
orbital fat
greater wing of sphenoid bone
optic nerve
ethmoid sinus
sphenoid sinus
cavernous sinus
dorsum sellae

nasal septum
lamina papyracea
medial rectus muscle
zygomatic bone
lateral rectus muscle
temporal lobe
anterior clinoid process
pituitary gland
posterior clinoid process
pons

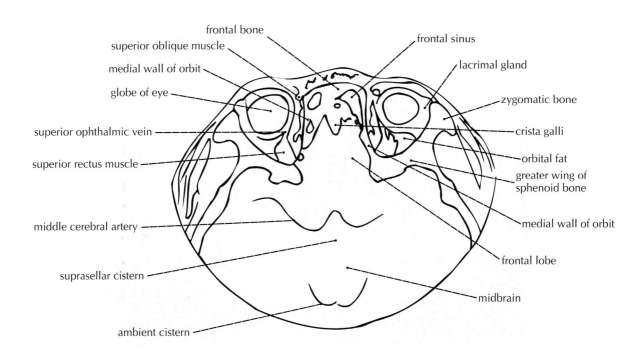

frontal bone
superior oblique muscle
medial wall of orbit
globe of eye
superior ophthalmic vein
superior rectus muscle
middle cerebral artery
suprasellar cistern
ambient cistern

frontal sinus
lacrimal gland
zygomatic bone
crista galli
orbital fat
greater wing of sphenoid bone
medial wall of orbit
frontal lobe
midbrain

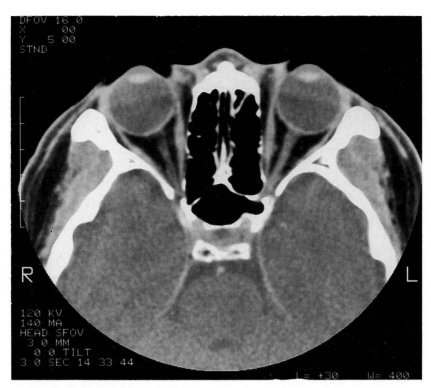

**1-29** Axial orbital CT scan (section 7 in Fig. 1-17).

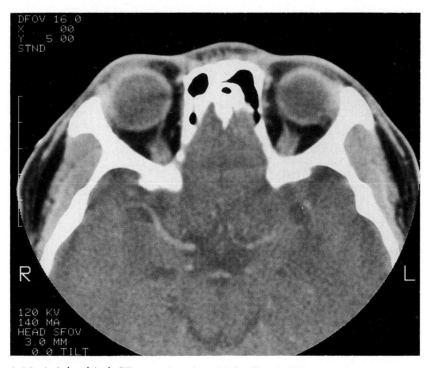

**1-30** Axial orbital CT scan (section 10 in Fig. 1-17).

# 1/Orbit, Coronal CT

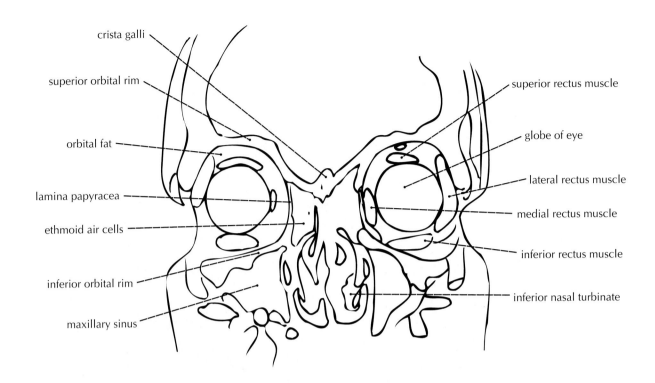

crista galli

superior orbital rim

orbital fat

lamina papyracea

ethmoid air cells

inferior orbital rim

maxillary sinus

superior rectus muscle

globe of eye

lateral rectus muscle

medial rectus muscle

inferior rectus muscle

inferior nasal turbinate

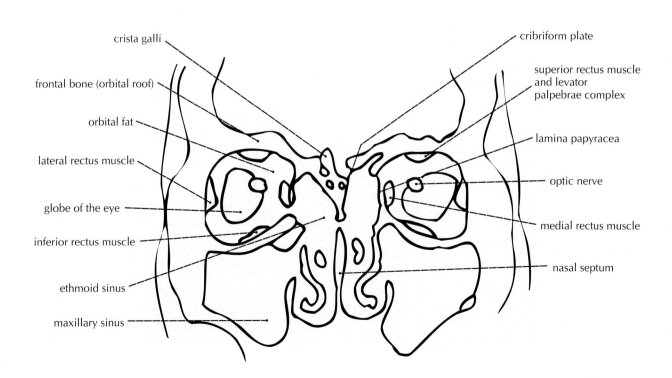

crista galli

frontal bone (orbital roof)

orbital fat

lateral rectus muscle

globe of the eye

inferior rectus muscle

ethmoid sinus

maxillary sinus

cribriform plate

superior rectus muscle
and levator
palpebrae complex

lamina papyracea

optic nerve

medial rectus muscle

nasal septum

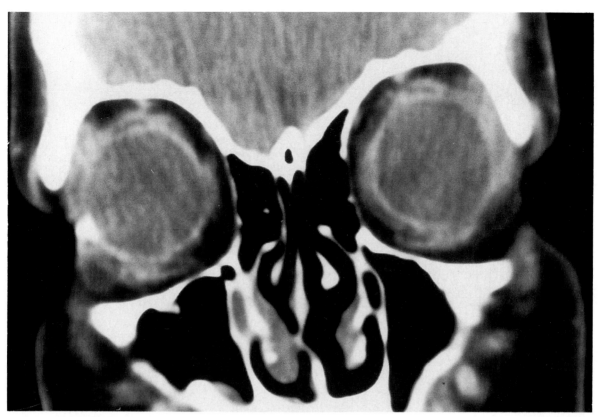

**1-31** Coronal CT scan through anterior orbit (section 4 in Fig. 1-23).

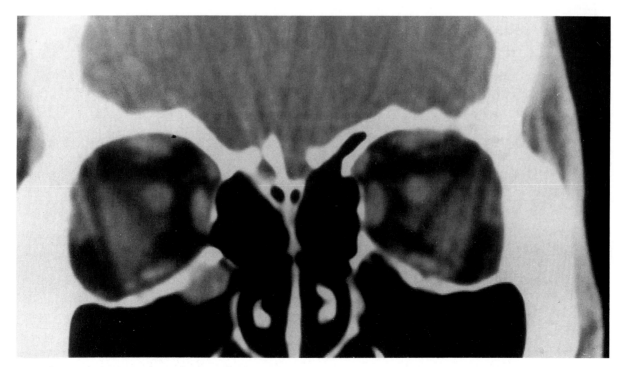

**1-32** Coronal CT scan through the orbit (section 6 in Fig. 1-23).

# 1/Orbit, Coronal CT

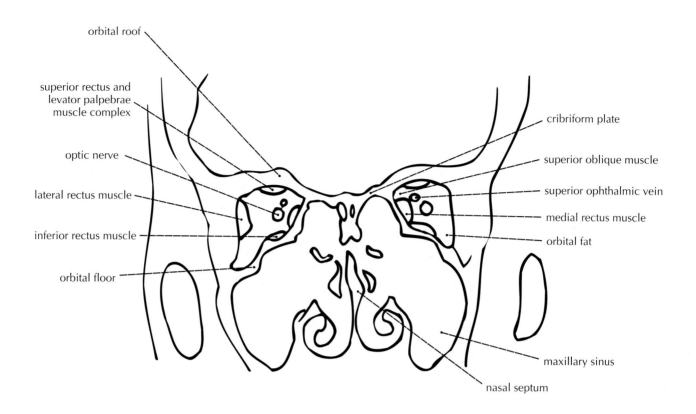

orbital roof

superior rectus and levator palpebrae muscle complex

optic nerve

lateral rectus muscle

inferior rectus muscle

orbital floor

cribriform plate

superior oblique muscle

superior ophthalmic vein

medial rectus muscle

orbital fat

maxillary sinus

nasal septum

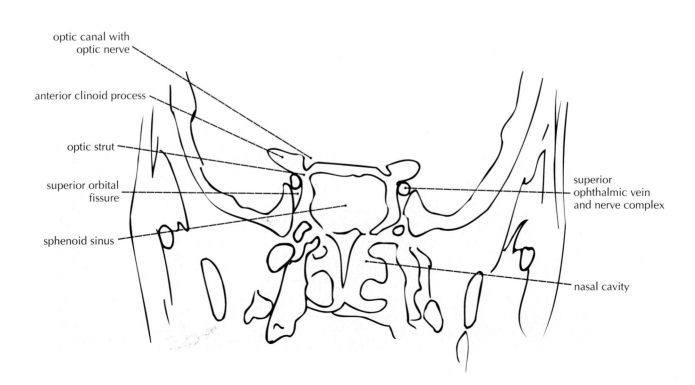

optic canal with optic nerve

anterior clinoid process

optic strut

superior orbital fissure

sphenoid sinus

superior ophthalmic vein and nerve complex

nasal cavity

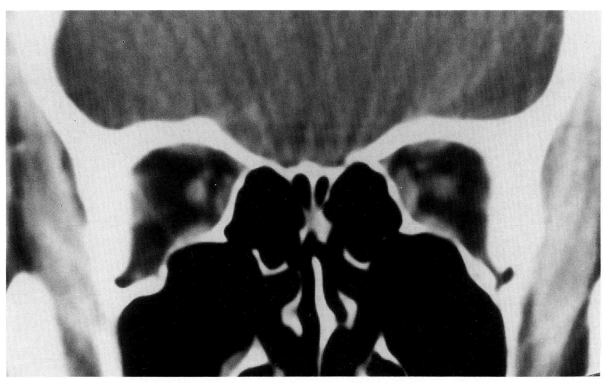

**1-33** Coronal CT scan through the orbit (section 10 in Fig. 1-23).

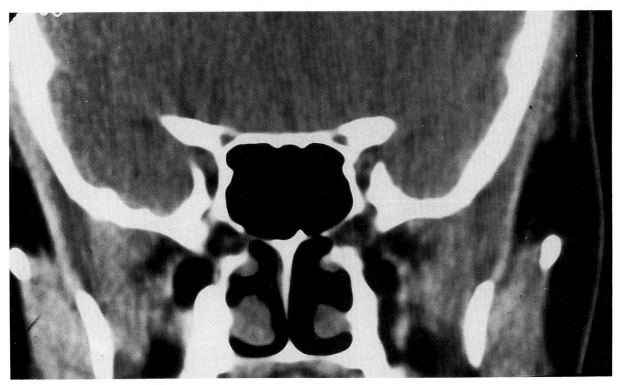

**1-34** Coronal CT scan through orbital apex (section 14 in Fig. 1-23).

# 1/Orbit, Coronal Scout and Axial MR

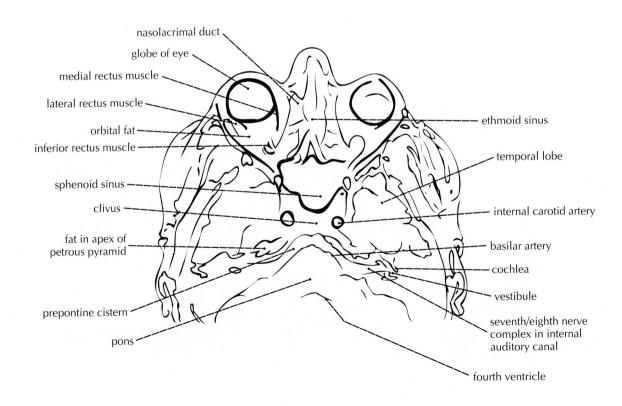

- nasolacrimal duct
- globe of eye
- medial rectus muscle
- lateral rectus muscle
- orbital fat
- inferior rectus muscle
- sphenoid sinus
- clivus
- fat in apex of petrous pyramid
- prepontine cistern
- pons
- ethmoid sinus
- temporal lobe
- internal carotid artery
- basilar artery
- cochlea
- vestibule
- seventh/eighth nerve complex in internal auditory canal
- fourth ventricle

# 1/Orbit, Coronal Scout and Axial MR

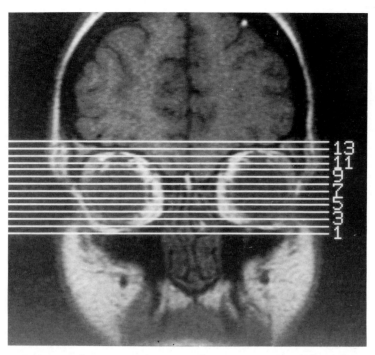

**1-35** Coronal MR scout image to demonstrate selected axial orbital MR sections.

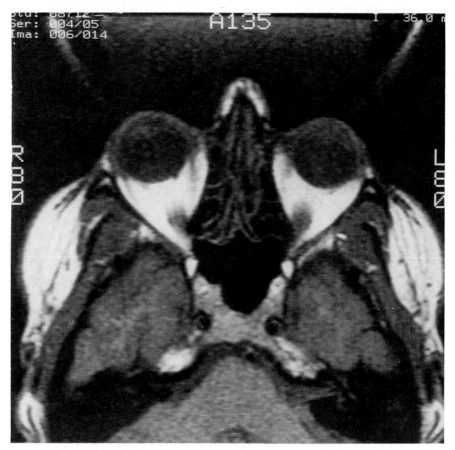

**1-36** Axial MR scan through lower orbit (600/20) (section 6 in Fig. 1-35).

# 1/Orbit, Axial MR

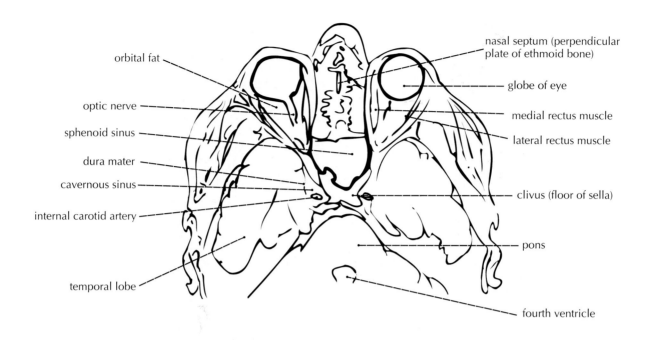

orbital fat

optic nerve

sphenoid sinus

dura mater

cavernous sinus

internal carotid artery

temporal lobe

nasal septum (perpendicular plate of ethmoid bone)

globe of eye

medial rectus muscle

lateral rectus muscle

clivus (floor of sella)

pons

fourth ventricle

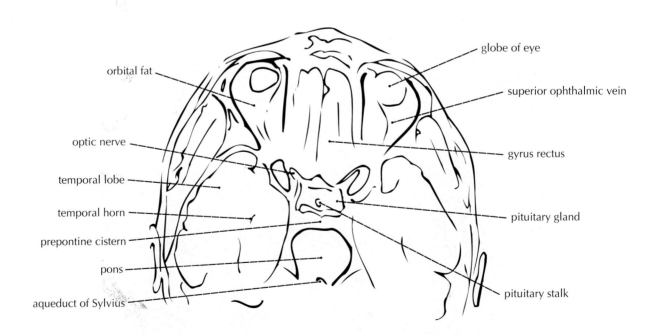

orbital fat

optic nerve

temporal lobe

temporal horn

prepontine cistern

pons

aqueduct of Sylvius

globe of eye

superior ophthalmic vein

gyrus rectus

pituitary gland

pituitary stalk

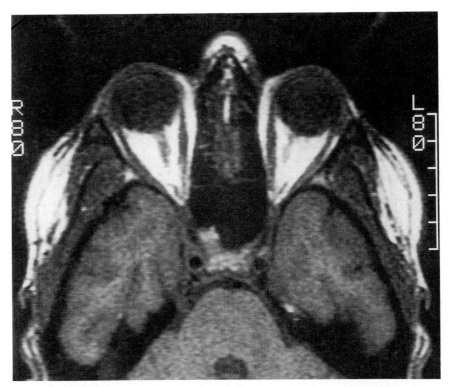

**1-37** Axial MR scan through midorbit (600/20) (section 8 in Fig. 1-35).

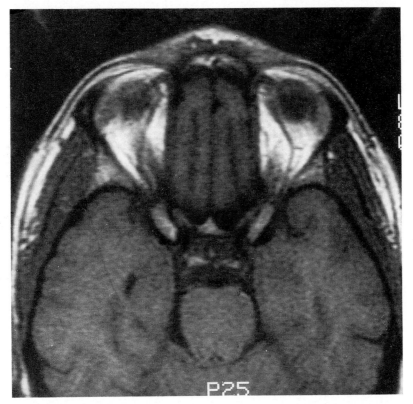

**1-38** Axial orbital MR scan (600/20) (section 11 in Fig. 1-35).

# 1/Orbit, Axial MR

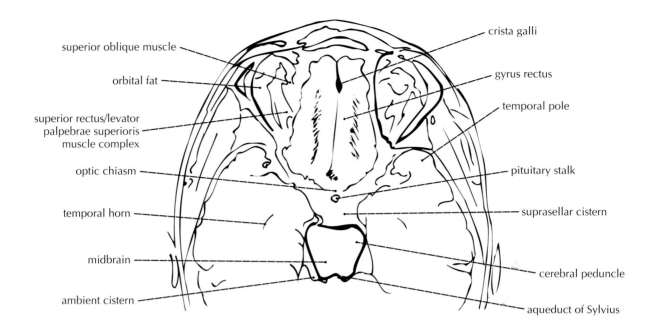

superior oblique muscle

orbital fat

superior rectus/levator
palpebrae superioris
muscle complex

optic chiasm

temporal horn

midbrain

ambient cistern

crista galli

gyrus rectus

temporal pole

pituitary stalk

suprasellar cistern

cerebral peduncle

aqueduct of Sylvius

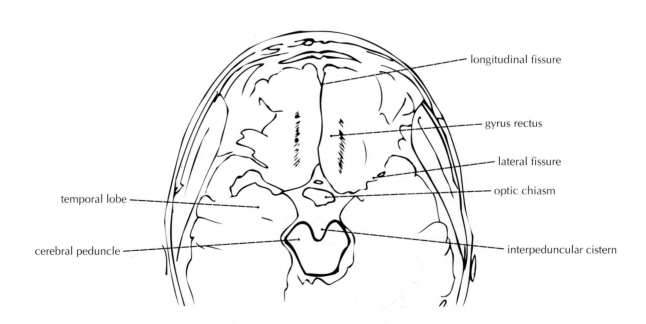

longitudinal fissure

gyrus rectus

lateral fissure

optic chiasm

temporal lobe

cerebral peduncle

interpeduncular cistern

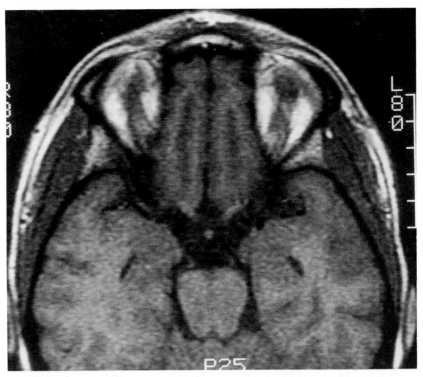

**1-39** Axial orbital MR scan (600/20) (section 12 in Fig. 1-35).

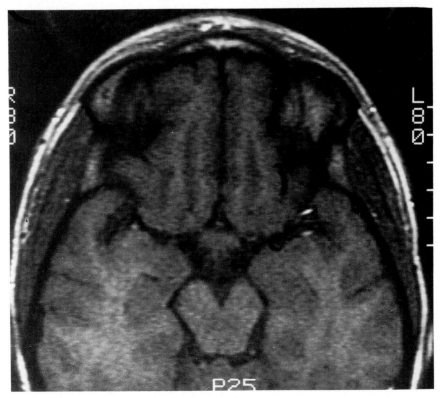

**1-40** Axial MR scan through upper orbit and low frontal lobes (600/20) (section 13 in Fig. 1-35).

# 1/Orbit, Sagittal Scout and Coronal MR

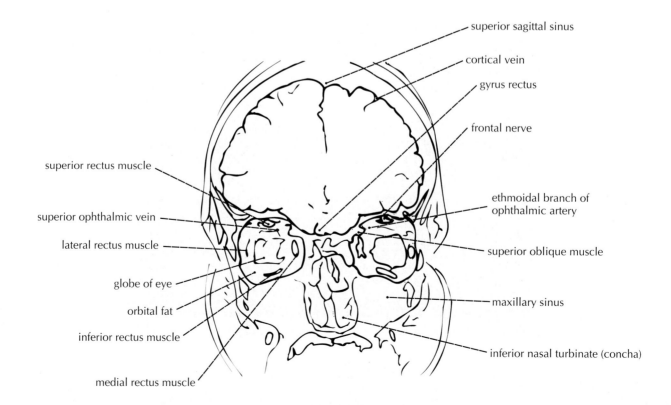

superior sagittal sinus

cortical vein

gyrus rectus

frontal nerve

superior rectus muscle

ethmoidal branch of
ophthalmic artery

superior ophthalmic vein

lateral rectus muscle

superior oblique muscle

globe of eye

orbital fat

maxillary sinus

inferior rectus muscle

inferior nasal turbinate (concha)

medial rectus muscle

# 1/Orbit, Sagittal Scout and Coronal MR

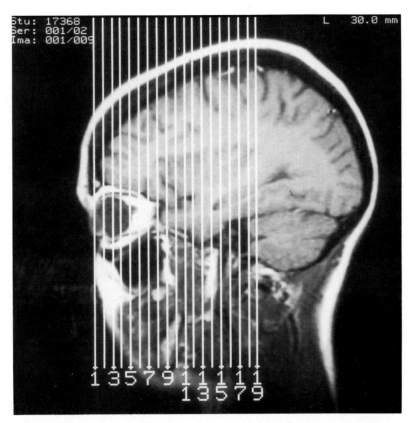

**1-41** Sagittal scout MR scan used to demonstrate the location of selected coronal MR scans of the orbit.

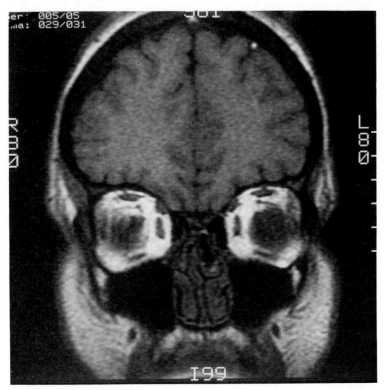

**1-42** Coronal MR scan through orbits (600/20) (section 4 in Fig. 1-41).

# 1/Orbit, Coronal MR

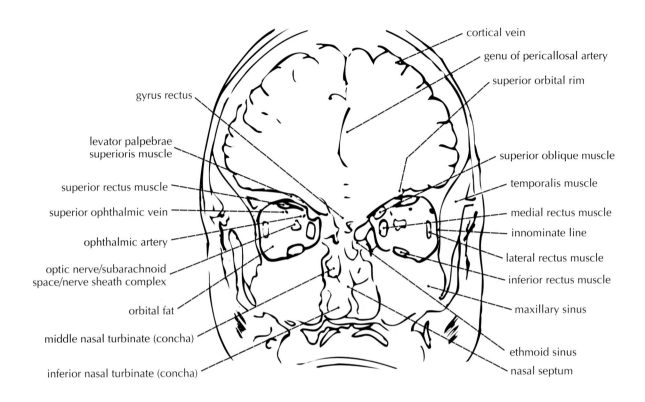

cortical vein

genu of pericallosal artery

superior orbital rim

gyrus rectus

levator palpebrae superioris muscle

superior oblique muscle

superior rectus muscle

temporalis muscle

superior ophthalmic vein

medial rectus muscle

ophthalmic artery

innominate line

optic nerve/subarachnoid space/nerve sheath complex

lateral rectus muscle

inferior rectus muscle

orbital fat

maxillary sinus

middle nasal turbinate (concha)

ethmoid sinus

inferior nasal turbinate (concha)

nasal septum

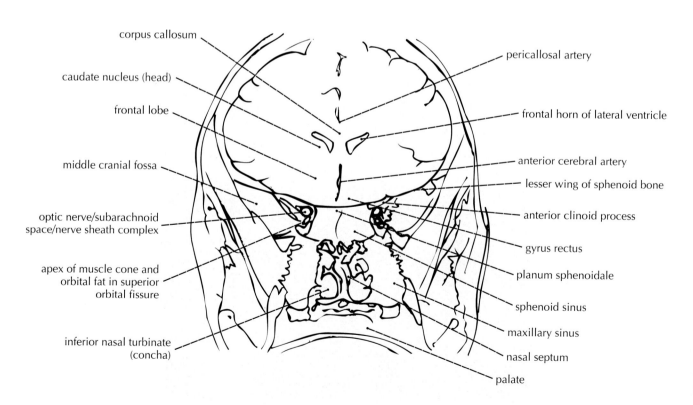

corpus callosum

pericallosal artery

caudate nucleus (head)

frontal lobe

frontal horn of lateral ventricle

middle cranial fossa

anterior cerebral artery

lesser wing of sphenoid bone

optic nerve/subarachnoid space/nerve sheath complex

anterior clinoid process

gyrus rectus

apex of muscle cone and orbital fat in superior orbital fissure

planum sphenoidale

sphenoid sinus

maxillary sinus

inferior nasal turbinate (concha)

nasal septum

palate

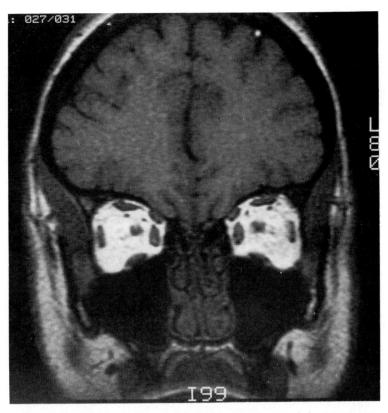

**1-43** Coronal MR scan through orbit (posterior to globe) (600/20). Section 7 in Fig. 1-41.

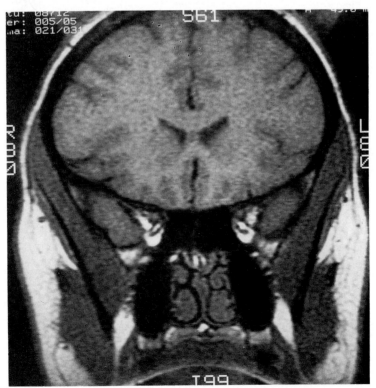

**1-44** Coronal MR scan through posterior orbit (600/20). Section 9 in Fig. 1-41.

# 1/Optic Chiasm and Pituitary Gland, Coronal MR

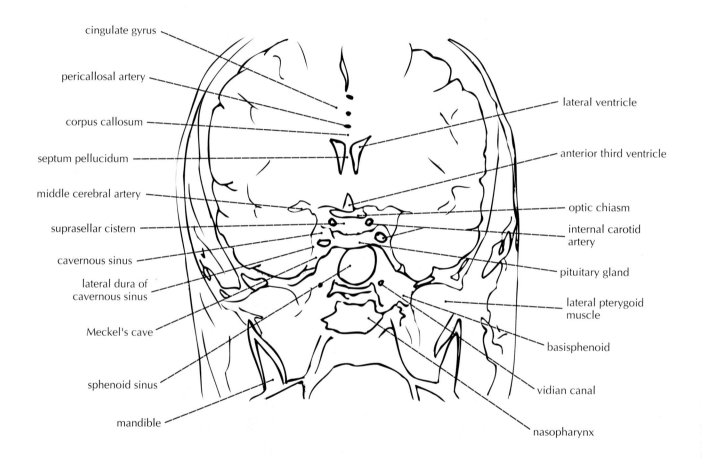

cingulate gyrus

pericallosal artery

corpus callosum

septum pellucidum

middle cerebral artery

suprasellar cistern

cavernous sinus

lateral dura of
cavernous sinus

Meckel's cave

sphenoid sinus

mandible

lateral ventricle

anterior third ventricle

optic chiasm

internal carotid
artery

pituitary gland

lateral pterygoid
muscle

basisphenoid

vidian canal

nasopharynx

# 1/Optic Chiasm and Pituitary Gland, Coronal MR

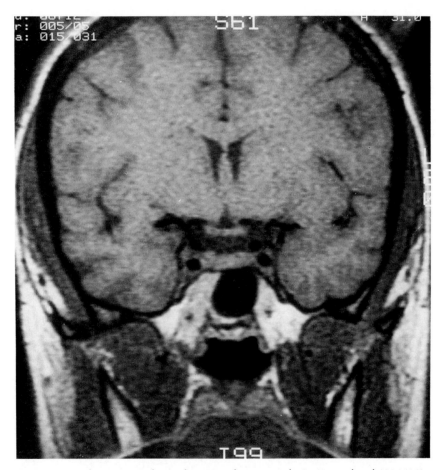

**1-45** Coronal MR scan through optic chiasm and pituitary gland (600/20). Section 12 in Fig. 1-41.

# 2/Brain, Head, Sella Turcica, and Temporal Bone □ Brain

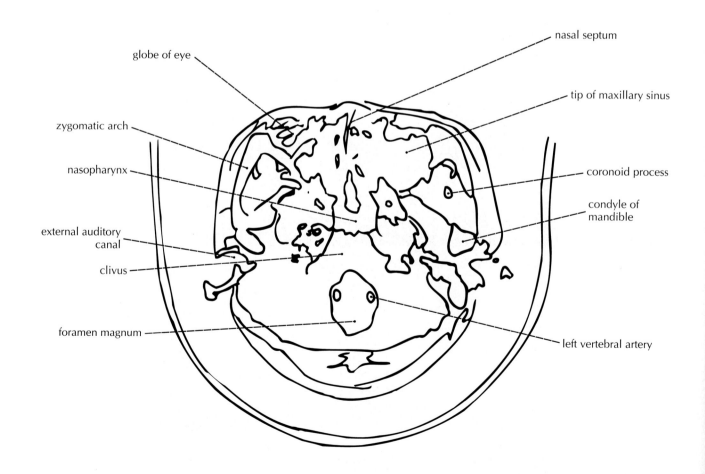

globe of eye

nasal septum

tip of maxillary sinus

zygomatic arch

nasopharynx

coronoid process

condyle of mandible

external auditory canal

clivus

foramen magnum

left vertebral artery

# 2/Brain, Sagittal Scout CT and Axial CT

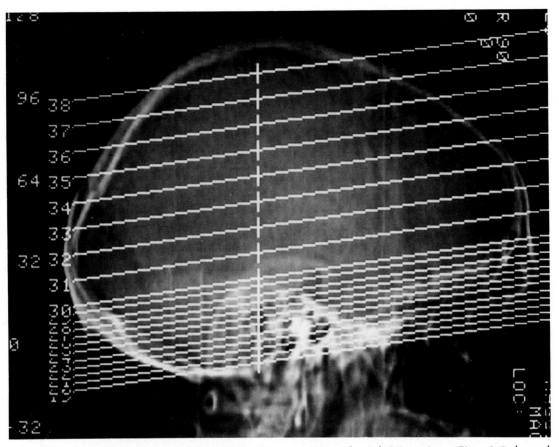

**2-1** Sagittal CT scout of the head used for demonstration of axial CT sections (Figs. 2-2 through 2-11).

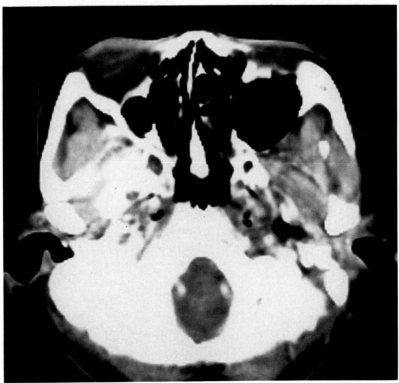

**2-2** Axial CT scan through foramen magnum (contrast-enhanced study). Section 19 in Fig. 2-1.

# 2/Brain, Axial CT

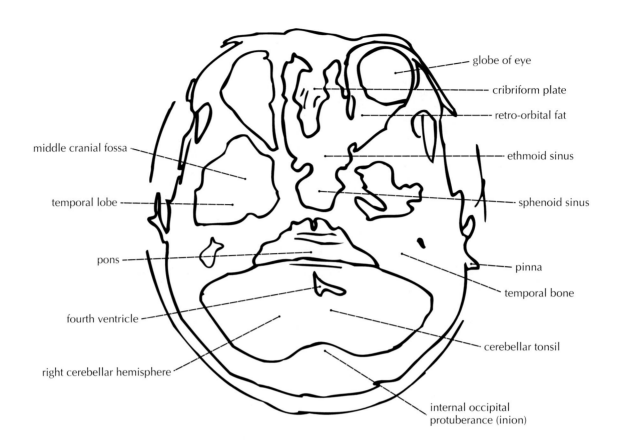

globe of eye

cribriform plate

retro-orbital fat

middle cranial fossa

ethmoid sinus

temporal lobe

sphenoid sinus

pons

pinna

temporal bone

fourth ventricle

cerebellar tonsil

right cerebellar hemisphere

internal occipital
protuberance (inion)

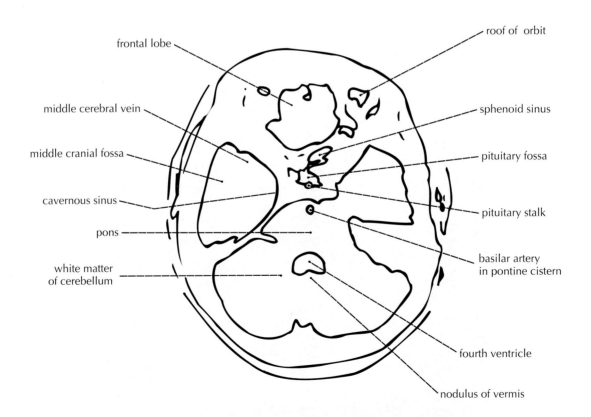

frontal lobe

roof of orbit

middle cerebral vein

sphenoid sinus

middle cranial fossa

pituitary fossa

cavernous sinus

pons

pituitary stalk

white matter
of cerebellum

basilar artery
in pontine cistern

fourth ventricle

nodulus of vermis

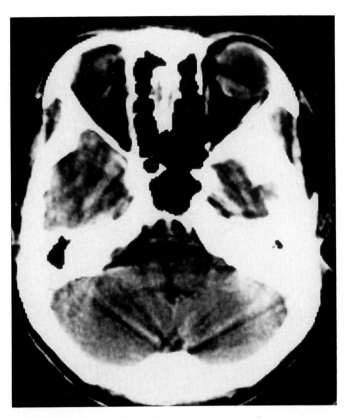

**2-3** Axial CT scan through lower posterior fossa (contrast-enhanced study). Section 25 in Fig. 2-1.

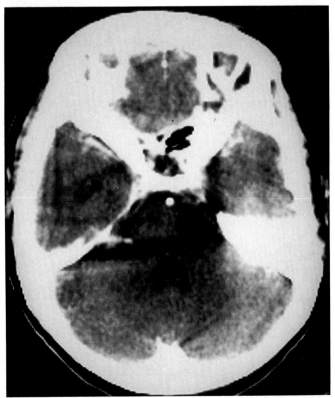

**2-4** Axial CT scan through fourth ventricle (contrast-enhanced study). Section 27 in Fig. 2-1.

# 2/Brain, Axial CT

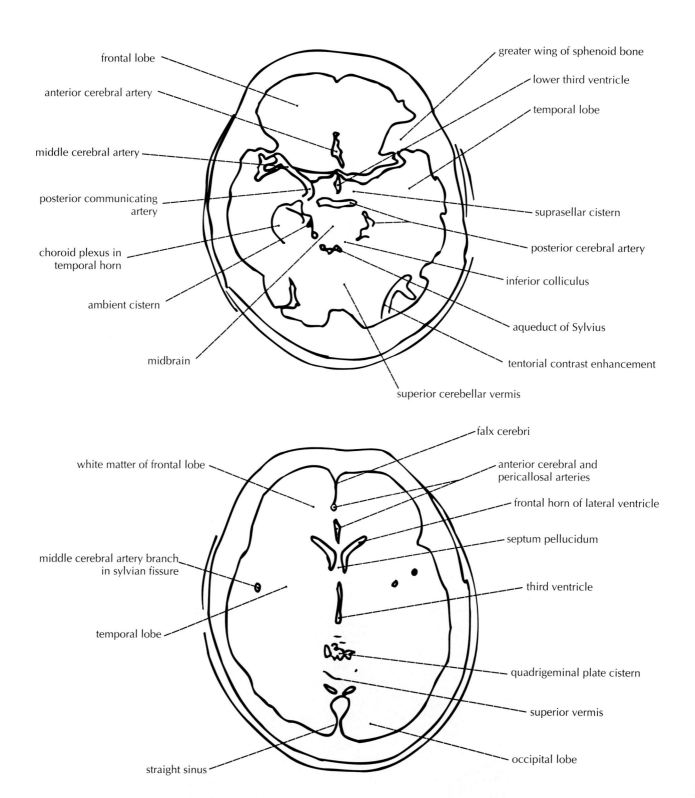

frontal lobe

anterior cerebral artery

middle cerebral artery

posterior communicating artery

choroid plexus in temporal horn

ambient cistern

midbrain

greater wing of sphenoid bone

lower third ventricle

temporal lobe

suprasellar cistern

posterior cerebral artery

inferior colliculus

aqueduct of Sylvius

tentorial contrast enhancement

superior cerebellar vermis

white matter of frontal lobe

middle cerebral artery branch in sylvian fissure

temporal lobe

straight sinus

falx cerebri

anterior cerebral and pericallosal arteries

frontal horn of lateral ventricle

septum pellucidum

third ventricle

quadrigeminal plate cistern

superior vermis

occipital lobe

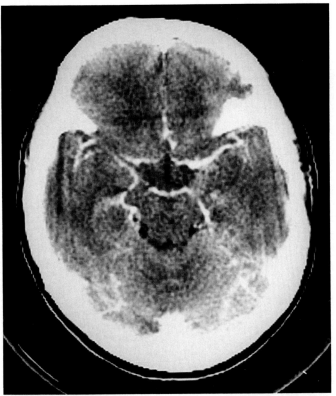

**2-5** Axial CT scan through midbrain (contrast-enhanced study). Section 30 in Fig. 2-1.

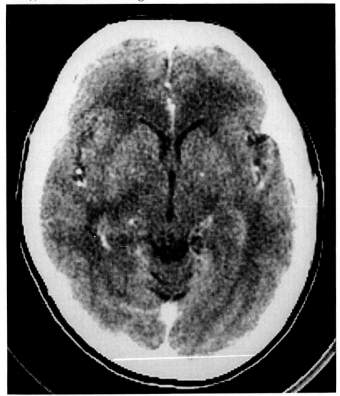

**2-6** Axial CT scan through third ventricle (contrast-enhanced study). Section 32 in Fig. 2-1.

# 2/Brain, Axial CT

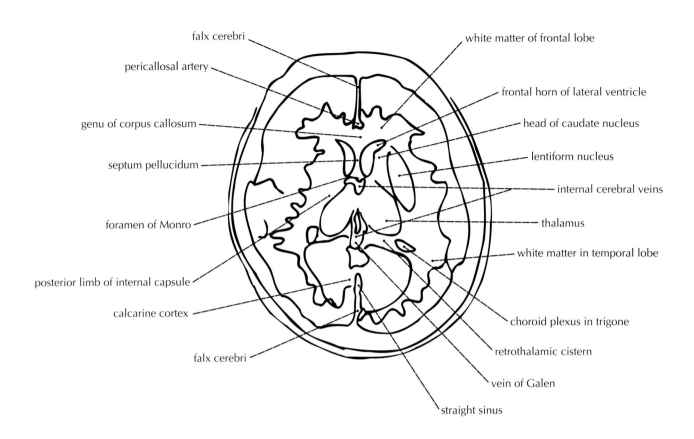

falx cerebri

pericallosal artery

genu of corpus callosum

septum pellucidum

foramen of Monro

posterior limb of internal capsule

calcarine cortex

falx cerebri

white matter of frontal lobe

frontal horn of lateral ventricle

head of caudate nucleus

lentiform nucleus

internal cerebral veins

thalamus

white matter in temporal lobe

choroid plexus in trigone

retrothalamic cistern

vein of Galen

straight sinus

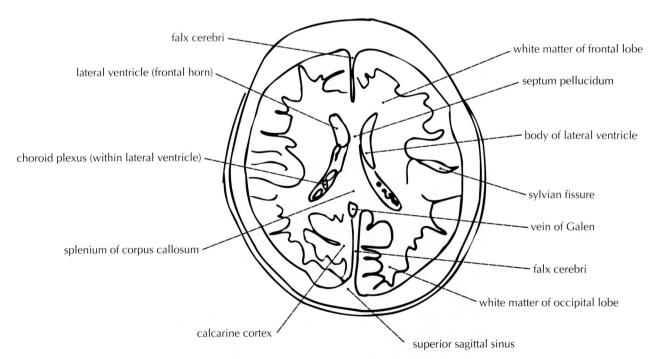

falx cerebri

lateral ventricle (frontal horn)

choroid plexus (within lateral ventricle)

splenium of corpus callosum

calcarine cortex

white matter of frontal lobe

septum pellucidum

body of lateral ventricle

sylvian fissure

vein of Galen

falx cerebri

white matter of occipital lobe

superior sagittal sinus

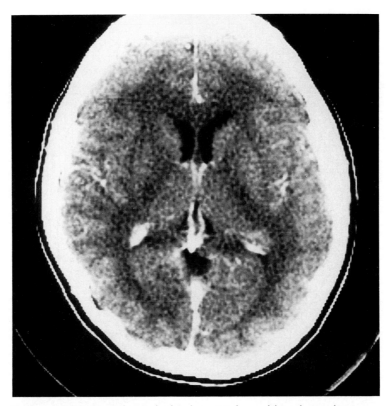

**2-7** Axial CT scan through third ventricle and basal ganglia (contrast-enhanced study). Section 33 in Fig. 2-1.

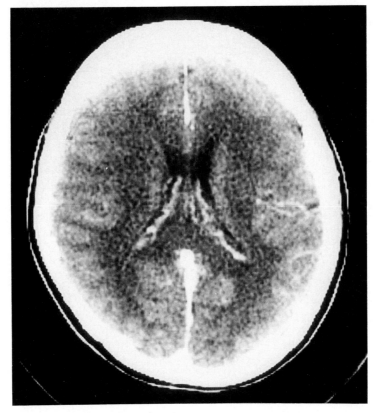

**2-8** Axial CT scan through bodies of lateral ventricles (contrast-enhanced study). Section 34 in Fig. 2-1.

# 2/Brain, Axial CT

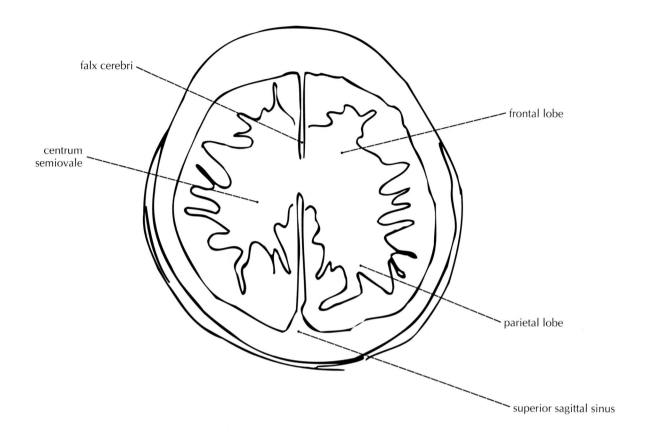

falx cerebri

frontal lobe

centrum
semiovale

parietal lobe

superior sagittal sinus

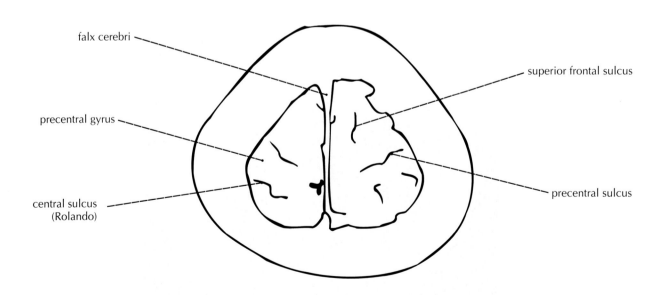

falx cerebri

superior frontal sulcus

precentral gyrus

central sulcus
(Rolando)

precentral sulcus

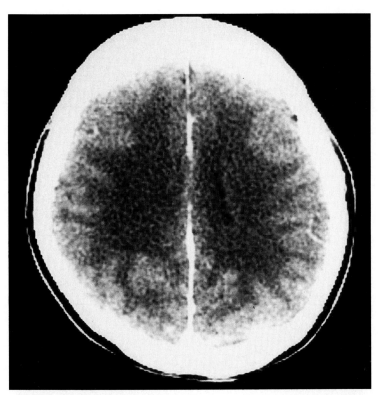

**2-9** Axial CT scan through centrum semiovale (contrast-enhanced study). Section 36 in Fig. 2-1.

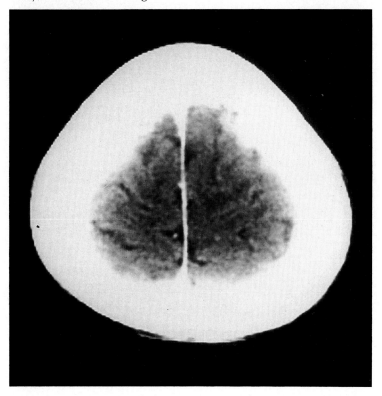

**2-10** Axial CT scan through vertex (contrast-enhanced study). Section 38 in Fig. 2-1.

# 2/Brain, Cisternography

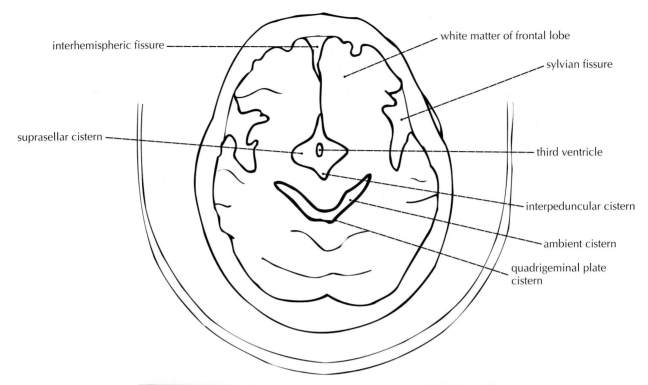

interhemispheric fissure ——————

white matter of frontal lobe

sylvian fissure

suprasellar cistern ——————

third ventricle

interpeduncular cistern

ambient cistern

quadrigeminal plate cistern

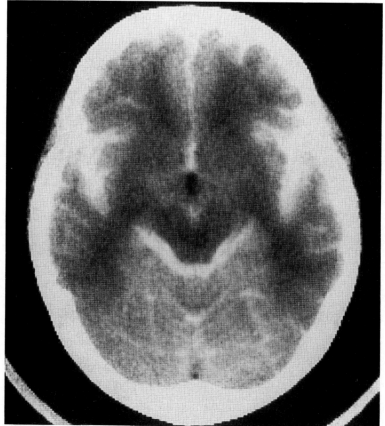

**2-11** Contrast cisternogram through suprasellar area. Section 31 in Fig. 2-1.

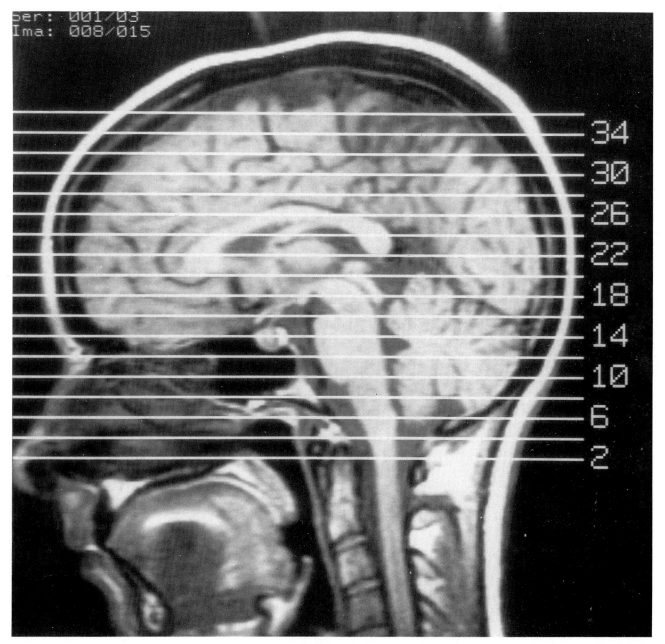

ber: 001/03
Ima: 008/015

34
30
26
22
18
14
10
6
2

**2-12** This sagittal scout MR scan is used to illustrate the locations of selected axial MR sections obtained with various techniques.

# 2/Brain, Axial MRI

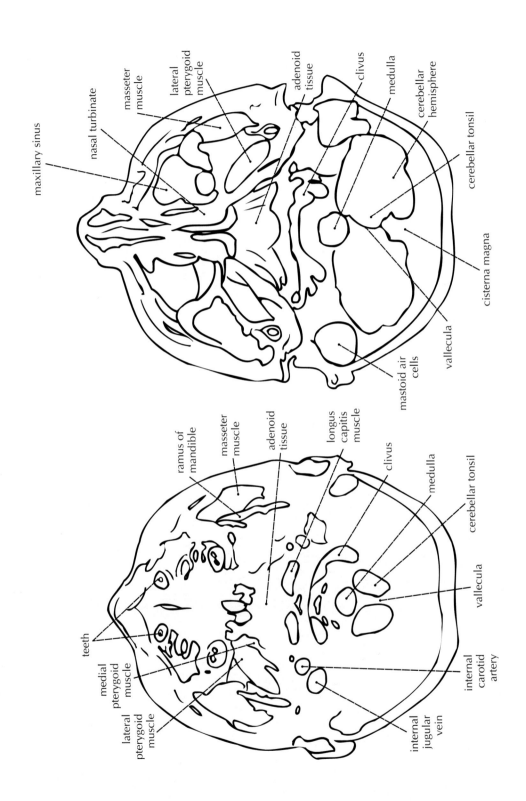

maxillary sinus

nasal turbinate

masseter muscle

lateral pterygoid muscle

adenoid tissue

clivus

medulla

cerebellar hemisphere

cerebellar tonsil

cisterna magna

vallecula

mastoid air cells

ramus of mandible

masseter muscle

adenoid tissue

longus capitis muscle

clivus

medulla

cerebellar tonsil

vallecula

internal carotid artery

internal jugular vein

teeth

medial pterygoid muscle

lateral pterygoid muscle

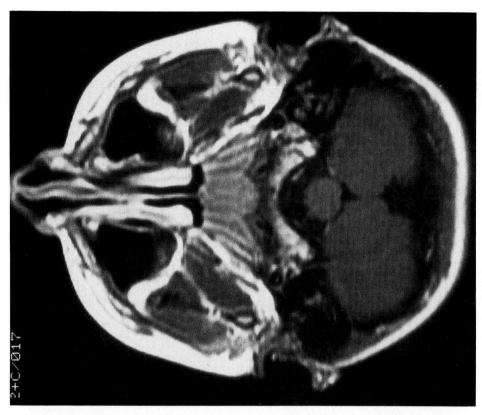

**2-14** Axial MR scan through posterior fossa (600/15). Contrast-enhanced study. Section 6 in Fig. 2-12.

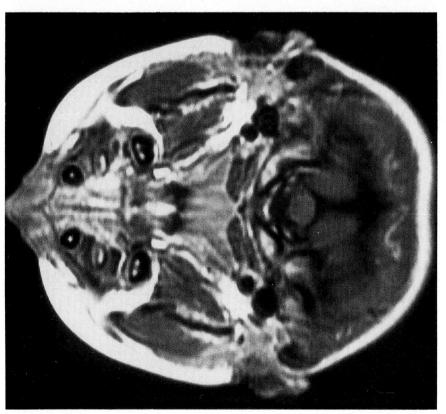

**2-13** Axial MR scan of the head (600/15). Contrast-enhanced study. Image between sections 4 and 6 in Fig. 2-12.

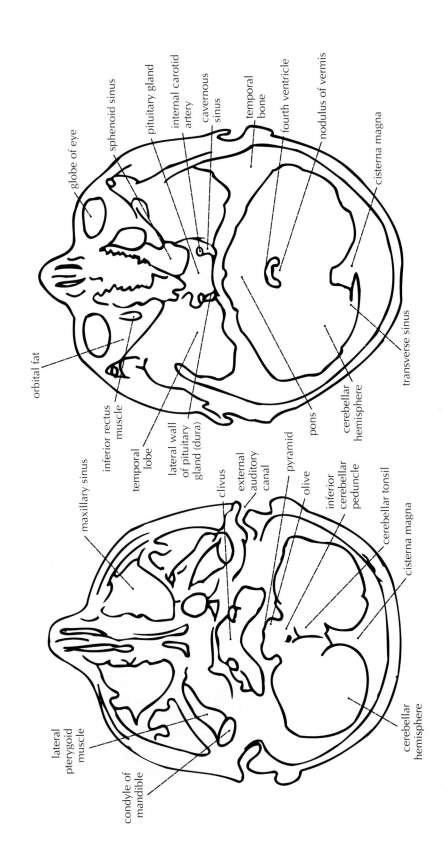

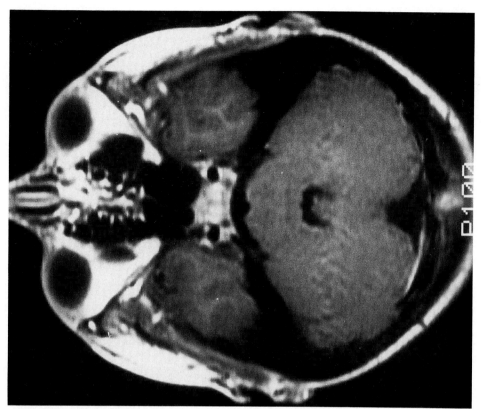

**2-16** Axial MR scan through fourth ventricle (600/15). Contrast-enhanced study. Section 12 in Fig. 2-12.

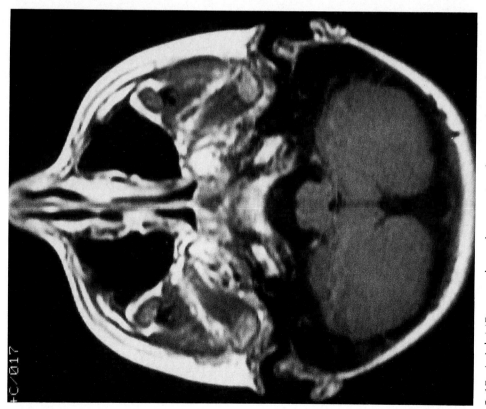

**2-15** Axial MR scan through posterior fossa and tonsils (600/15). Contrast-enhanced study. Section 8 in Fig. 2-12.

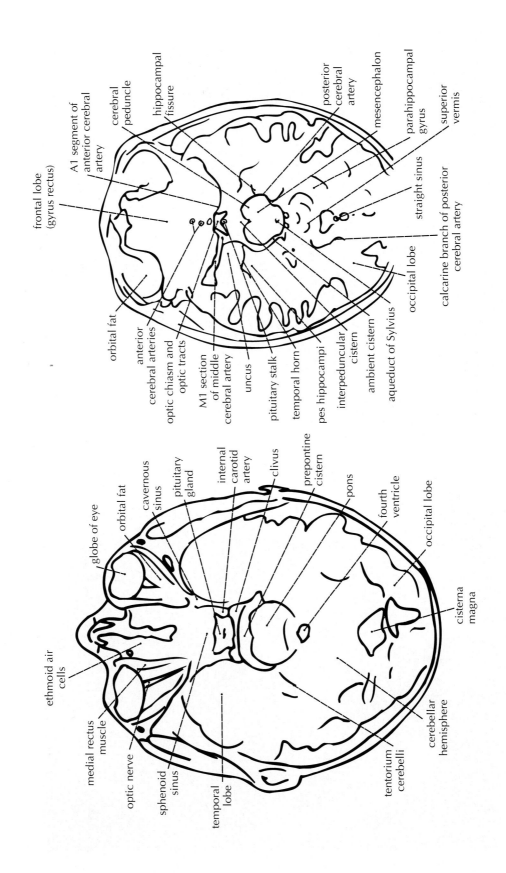

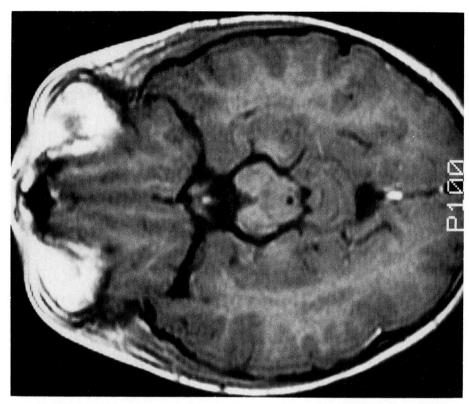

**2-18** Axial MR scan through suprasellar cistern (600/15). Contrast-enhanced study. Section 16 in Fig. 2-12.

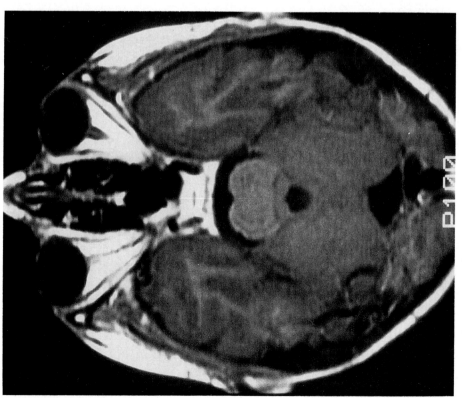

**2-17** Axial MR scan through pons (600/15). Contrast-enhanced study. Section 14 in Fig. 2-12.

# 2/Brain, Axial MRI

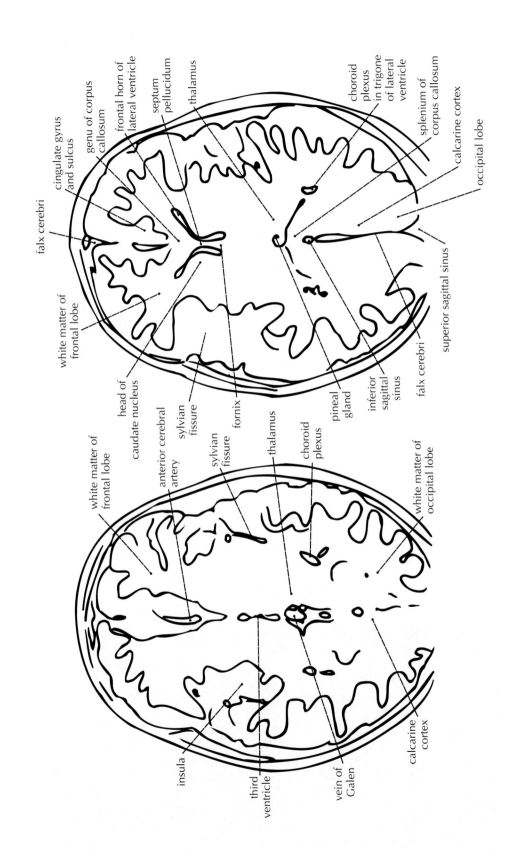

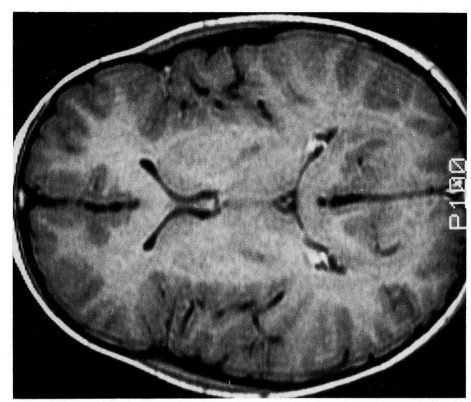

**2-20** Axial MR scan through lateral ventricles (600/15). Contrast-enhanced study. Section 22 in Fig. 2-12.

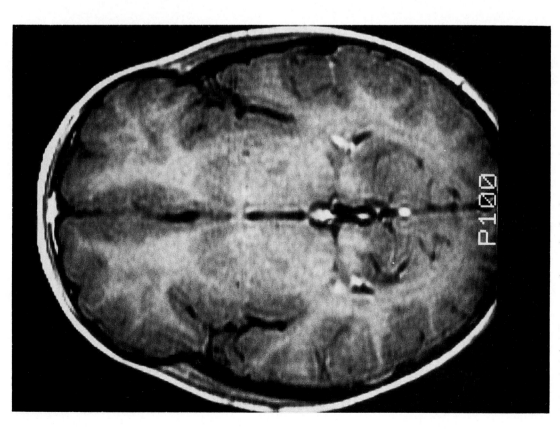

**2-19** Axial MR scan through third ventricle (600/15). Contrast-enhanced study. Section 20 in Fig. 2-12.

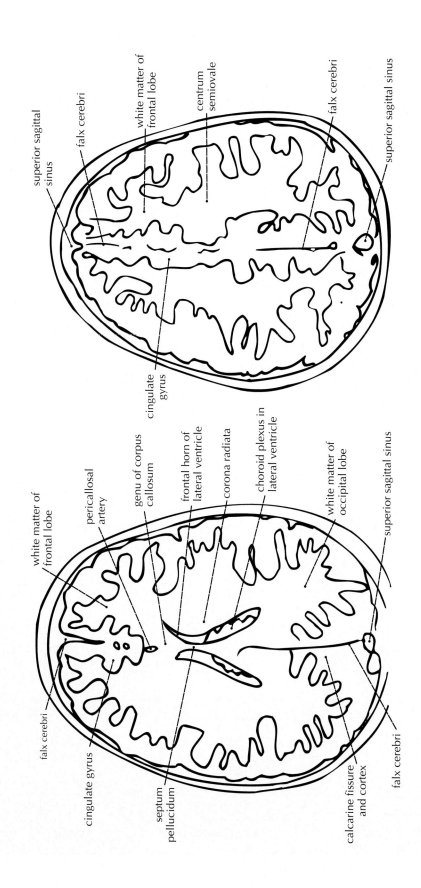

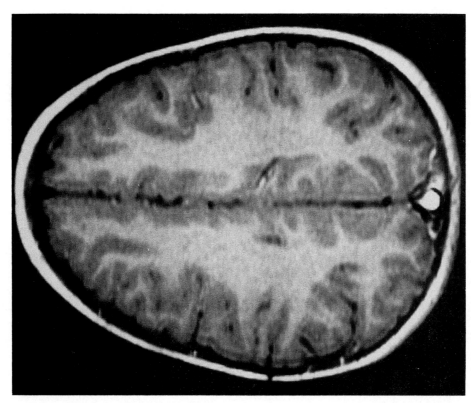

**2-22** Axial MR scan through centrum semiovale (600/15). Contrast-enhanced study. Section 26 in Fig. 2-12.

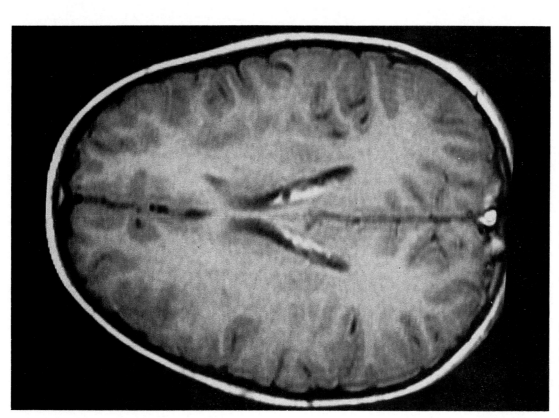

**2-21** Axial MR scan through lateral ventricles (600/15). Contrast-enhanced study. Section 24 in Fig. 2-12.

# 2/Brain, Axial MRI

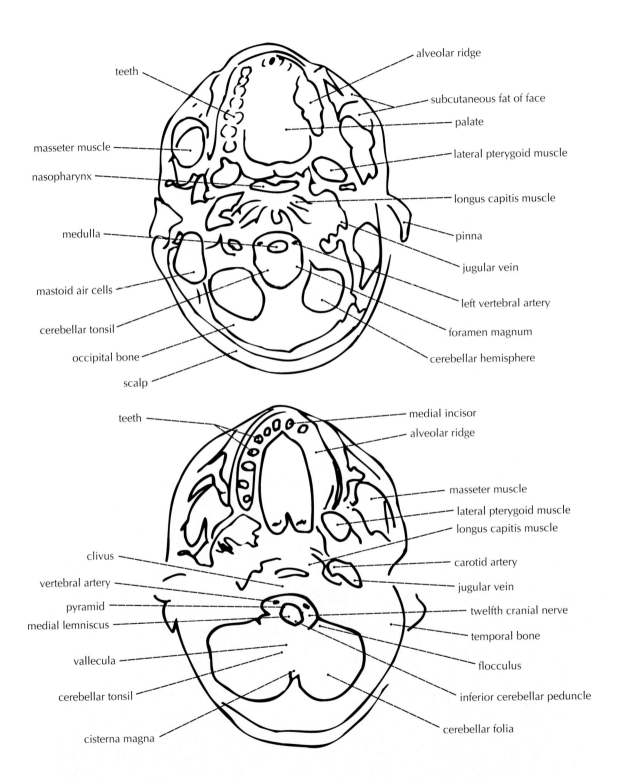

teeth

alveolar ridge

subcutaneous fat of face

palate

masseter muscle

lateral pterygoid muscle

nasopharynx

longus capitis muscle

medulla

pinna

jugular vein

mastoid air cells

left vertebral artery

cerebellar tonsil

foramen magnum

occipital bone

cerebellar hemisphere

scalp

teeth

medial incisor

alveolar ridge

masseter muscle

lateral pterygoid muscle

longus capitis muscle

clivus

carotid artery

vertebral artery

jugular vein

pyramid

twelfth cranial nerve

medial lemniscus

temporal bone

vallecula

flocculus

cerebellar tonsil

inferior cerebellar peduncle

cisterna magna

cerebellar folia

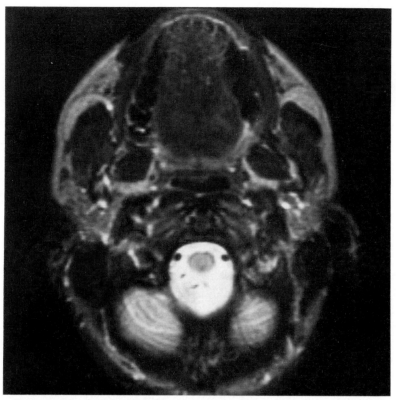

**2-23** Axial MR scan through foramen magnum and lower posterior fossa (2000/90). Section 4 in Fig. 2-12.

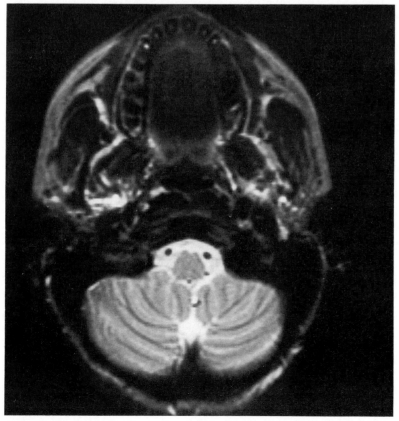

**2-24** Axial MR scan through posterior fossa (2000/90). Section 6 in Fig. 2-12.

# 2/Brain, Axial MR

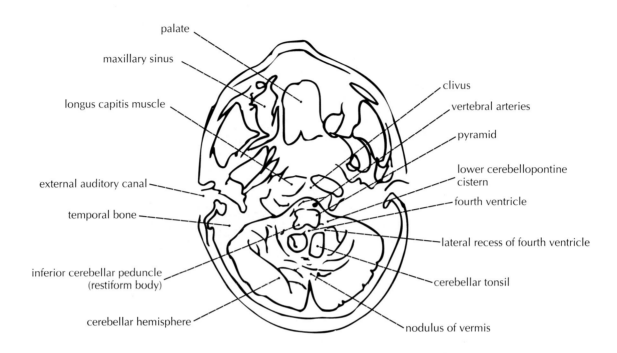

palate

maxillary sinus

longus capitis muscle

external auditory canal

temporal bone

inferior cerebellar peduncle
(restiform body)

cerebellar hemisphere

clivus

vertebral arteries

pyramid

lower cerebellopontine
cistern

fourth ventricle

lateral recess of fourth ventricle

cerebellar tonsil

nodulus of vermis

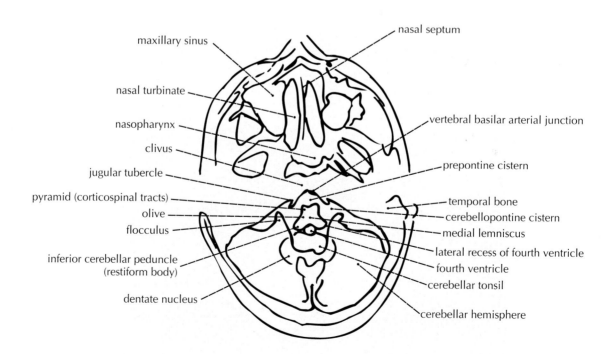

maxillary sinus

nasal turbinate

nasopharynx

clivus

jugular tubercle

pyramid (corticospinal tracts)

olive

flocculus

inferior cerebellar peduncle
(restiform body)

dentate nucleus

nasal septum

vertebral basilar arterial junction

prepontine cistern

temporal bone

cerebellopontine cistern

medial lemniscus

lateral recess of fourth ventricle

fourth ventricle

cerebellar tonsil

cerebellar hemisphere

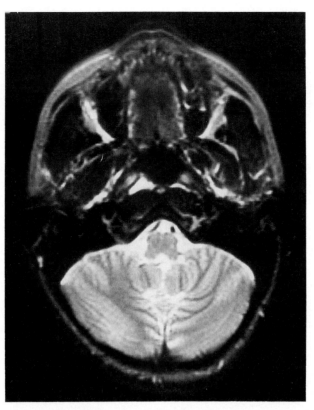

**2-25** Axial MR scan through lower fourth ventricle and medulla (2000/90). Section 8 in Fig. 2-12.

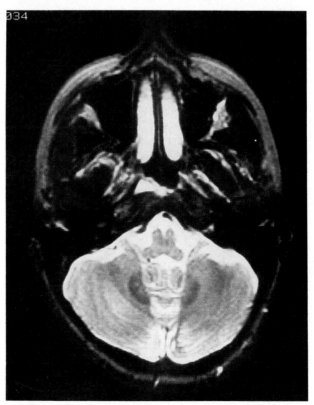

**2-26** Axial MR scan through lower fourth ventricle and medulla (2000/90). Section 10 in Fig. 2-12.

# 2/Brain, Axial MRI

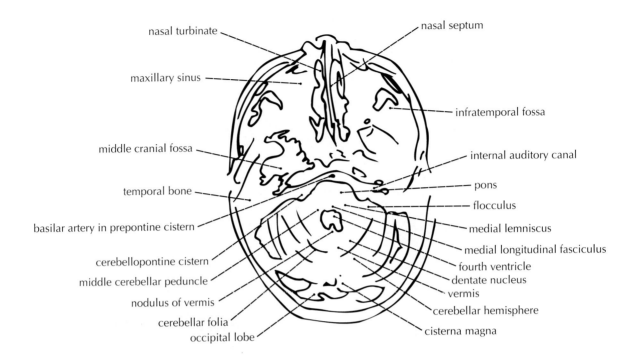

nasal turbinate
nasal septum
maxillary sinus
infratemporal fossa
middle cranial fossa
internal auditory canal
temporal bone
pons
flocculus
basilar artery in prepontine cistern
medial lemniscus
medial longitudinal fasciculus
cerebellopontine cistern
fourth ventricle
middle cerebellar peduncle
dentate nucleus
nodulus of vermis
vermis
cerebellar folia
cerebellar hemisphere
occipital lobe
cisterna magna

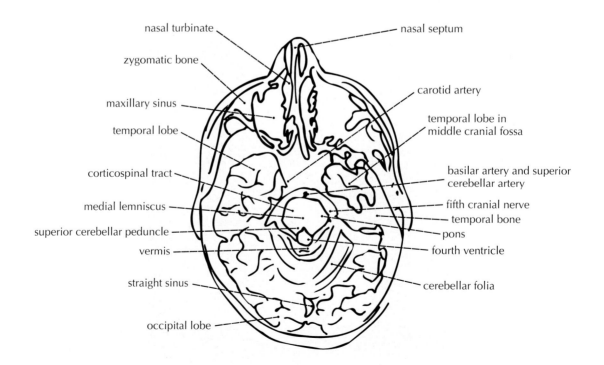

nasal turbinate
nasal septum
zygomatic bone
carotid artery
maxillary sinus
temporal lobe in middle cranial fossa
temporal lobe
corticospinal tract
basilar artery and superior cerebellar artery
medial lemniscus
fifth cranial nerve
temporal bone
superior cerebellar peduncle
pons
vermis
fourth ventricle
straight sinus
cerebellar folia
occipital lobe

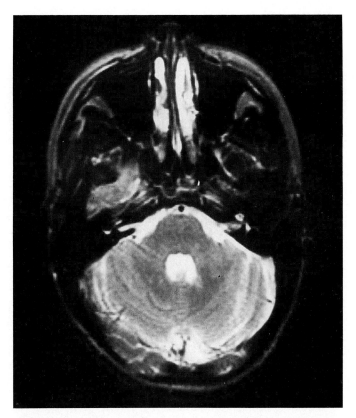

**2-27** Axial MR scan through fourth ventricle (2000/90). Section 12 in Fig. 2-12.

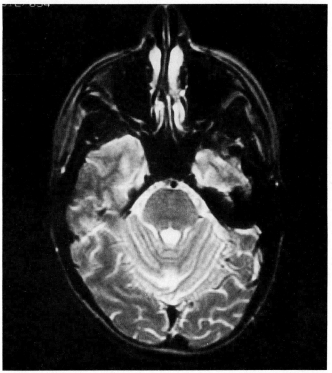

**2-28** Axial MR scan through fourth ventricle (2000/90). Section 14 in Fig. 2-12.

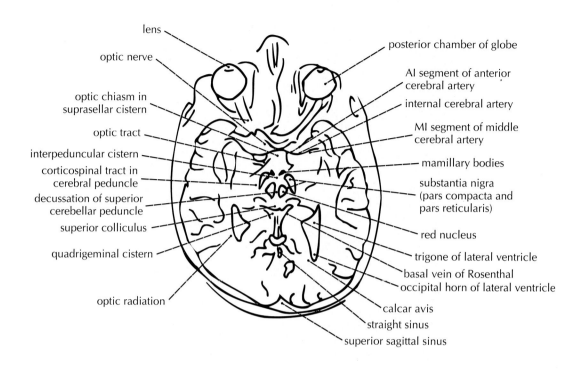

lens

optic nerve

optic chiasm in
suprasellar cistern

optic tract

interpeduncular cistern

corticospinal tract in
cerebral peduncle

decussation of superior
cerebellar peduncle

superior colliculus

quadrigeminal cistern

optic radiation

posterior chamber of globe

AI segment of anterior
cerebral artery

internal cerebral artery

MI segment of middle
cerebral artery

mamillary bodies

substantia nigra
(pars compacta and
pars reticularis)

red nucleus

trigone of lateral ventricle

basal vein of Rosenthal

occipital horn of lateral ventricle

calcar avis

straight sinus

superior sagittal sinus

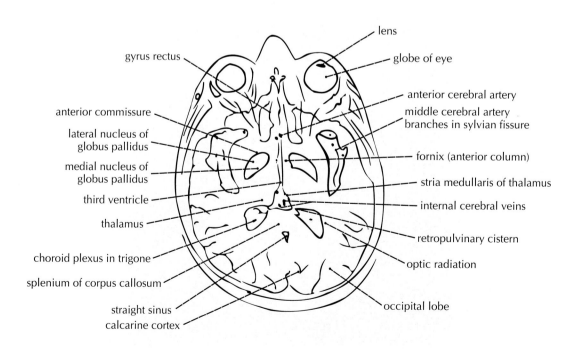

lens

gyrus rectus

globe of eye

anterior commissure

anterior cerebral artery

middle cerebral artery
branches in sylvian fissure

lateral nucleus of
globus pallidus

medial nucleus of
globus pallidus

third ventricle

thalamus

choroid plexus in trigone

splenium of corpus callosum

straight sinus

calcarine cortex

fornix (anterior column)

stria medullaris of thalamus

internal cerebral veins

retropulvinary cistern

optic radiation

occipital lobe

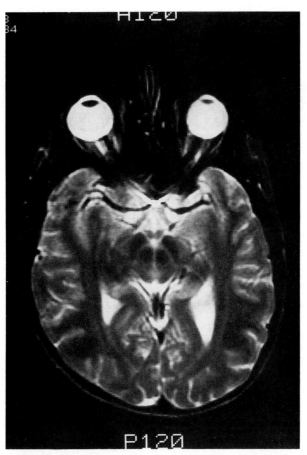

**2-29** Axial MR scan through midbrain (2000/90). Section 16 in Fig. 2-12.

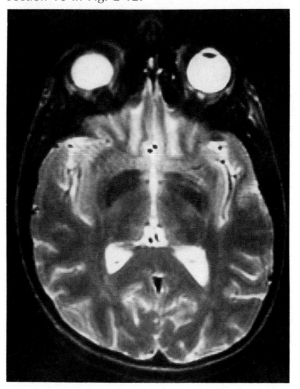

**2-30** Axial MR scan through third ventricle (2000/ 90). Section 20 in Fig. 2-12.

# 2/Brain, Axial MRI

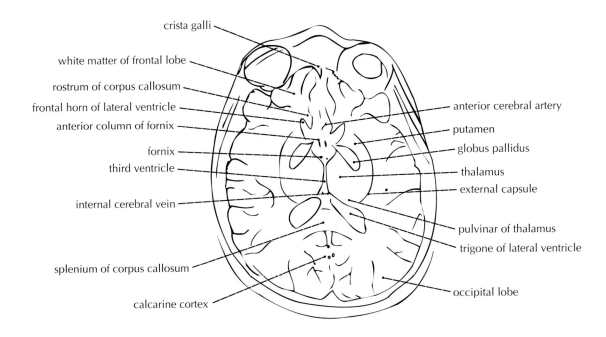

crista galli

white matter of frontal lobe

rostrum of corpus callosum

frontal horn of lateral ventricle

anterior column of fornix

fornix

third ventricle

internal cerebral vein

splenium of corpus callosum

calcarine cortex

anterior cerebral artery

putamen

globus pallidus

thalamus

external capsule

pulvinar of thalamus

trigone of lateral ventricle

occipital lobe

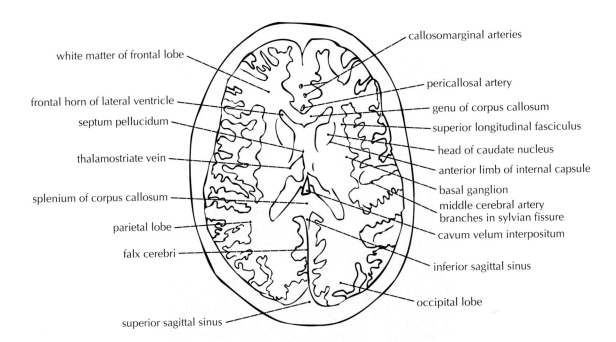

callosomarginal arteries

white matter of frontal lobe

frontal horn of lateral ventricle

septum pellucidum

thalamostriate vein

splenium of corpus callosum

parietal lobe

falx cerebri

superior sagittal sinus

pericallosal artery

genu of corpus callosum

superior longitudinal fasciculus

head of caudate nucleus

anterior limb of internal capsule

basal ganglion

middle cerebral artery branches in sylvian fissure

cavum velum interpositum

inferior sagittal sinus

occipital lobe

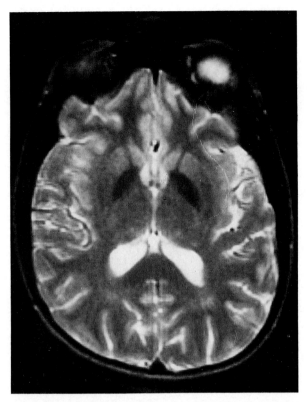

**2-31** Axial MR scan through third ventricle (2000/90). Section 22 in Fig. 2-12.

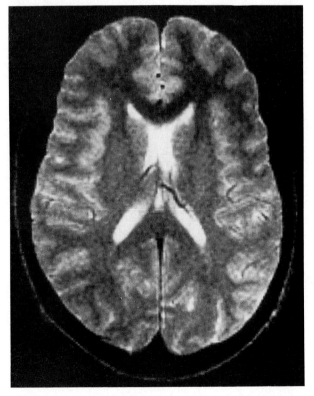

**2-32** Axial MR scan through lateral ventricles (2000/90). Section 24 in Fig. 2-12.

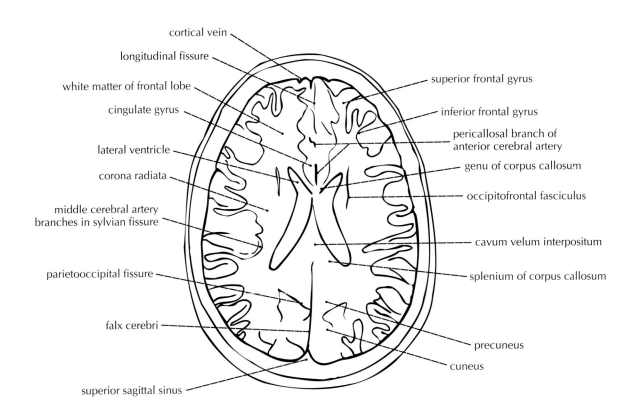

cortical vein
longitudinal fissure
white matter of frontal lobe
cingulate gyrus
lateral ventricle
corona radiata
middle cerebral artery
branches in sylvian fissure
parietooccipital fissure
falx cerebri
superior sagittal sinus

superior frontal gyrus
inferior frontal gyrus
pericallosal branch of
anterior cerebral artery
genu of corpus callosum
occipitofrontal fasciculus
cavum velum interpositum
splenium of corpus callosum
precuneus
cuneus

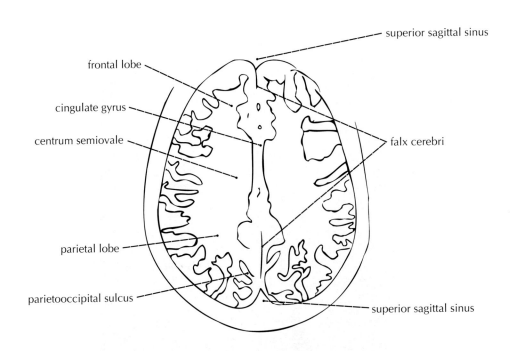

frontal lobe
cingulate gyrus
centrum semiovale
parietal lobe
parietooccipital sulcus

superior sagittal sinus
falx cerebri
superior sagittal sinus

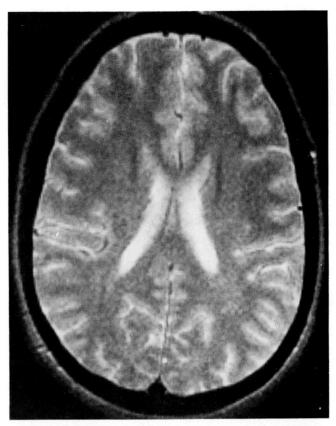

**2-33** Axial MR scan through lateral ventricles (2000/90). Section 26 in Fig. 2-12.

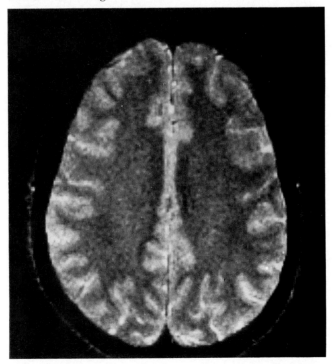

**2-34** Axial MR scan through parietal lobe above the ventricles (2000/90). Section 28 in Fig. 2-12.

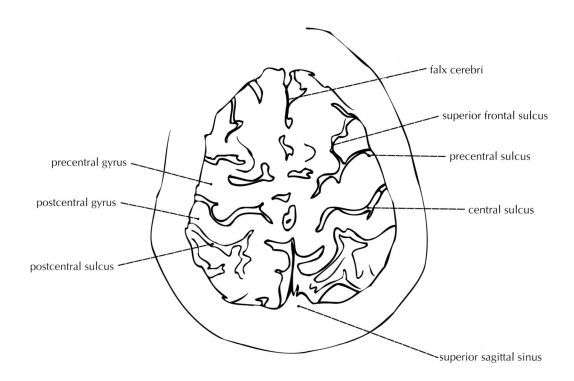

falx cerebri

superior frontal sulcus

precentral sulcus

central sulcus

superior sagittal sinus

precentral gyrus

postcentral gyrus

postcentral sulcus

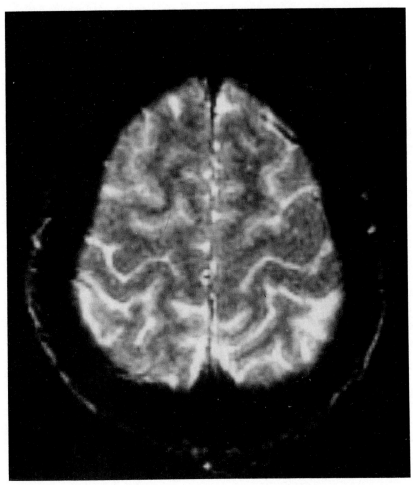

**2-35** Axial MR scan through vertex (2000/90). Section 34 in Fig. 2-12.

# 2/Brain, Sagittal Scout MRI and Coronal MRI

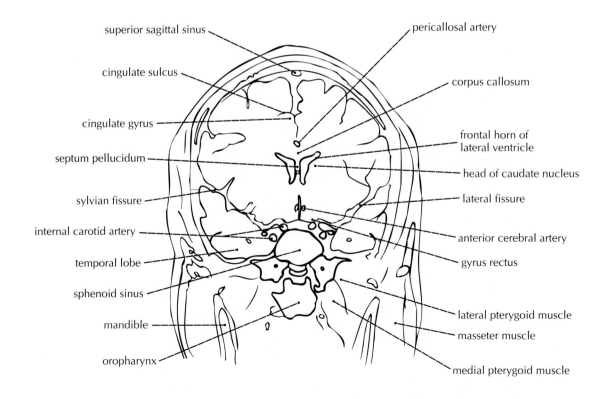

superior sagittal sinus

cingulate sulcus

cingulate gyrus

septum pellucidum

sylvian fissure

internal carotid artery

temporal lobe

sphenoid sinus

mandible

oropharynx

pericallosal artery

corpus callosum

frontal horn of lateral ventricle

head of caudate nucleus

lateral fissure

anterior cerebral artery

gyrus rectus

lateral pterygoid muscle

masseter muscle

medial pterygoid muscle

# 2/Brain, Sagittal Scout MRI and Coronal MRI

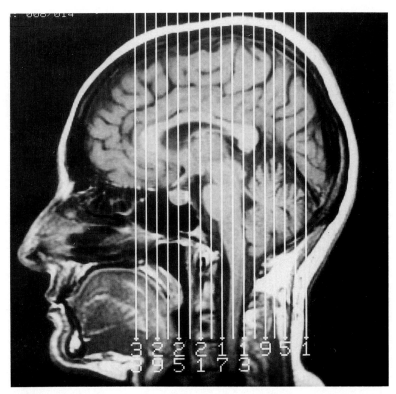

**2-36** Sagittal MR scout scan demonstrating coronal MR sections obtained with various techniques (Fig. 2-37 through 2-49).

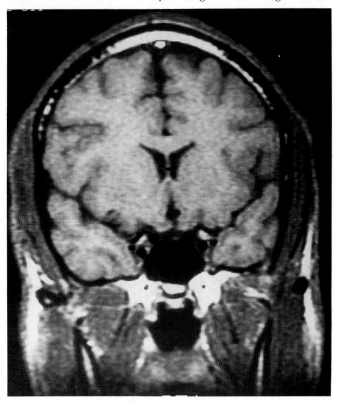

**2-37** Coronal MR scan through frontal lobes (800/20). Section 29 in Fig. 2-36.

# 2/Brain, Coronal MRI

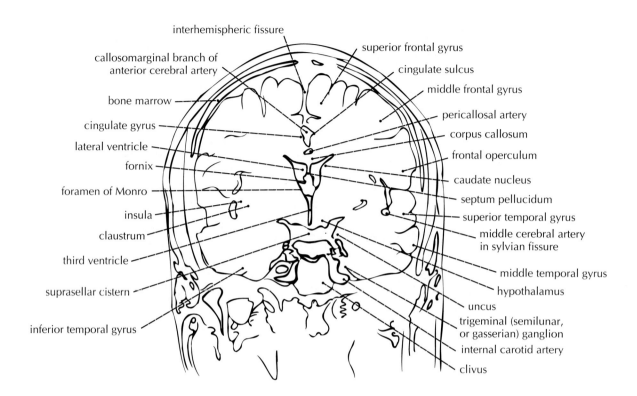

interhemispheric fissure

superior frontal gyrus

callosomarginal branch of anterior cerebral artery

cingulate sulcus

middle frontal gyrus

bone marrow

pericallosal artery

cingulate gyrus

corpus callosum

lateral ventricle

frontal operculum

fornix

caudate nucleus

foramen of Monro

septum pellucidum

insula

superior temporal gyrus

claustrum

middle cerebral artery in sylvian fissure

third ventricle

middle temporal gyrus

suprasellar cistern

hypothalamus

uncus

inferior temporal gyrus

trigeminal (semilunar, or gasserian) ganglion

internal carotid artery

clivus

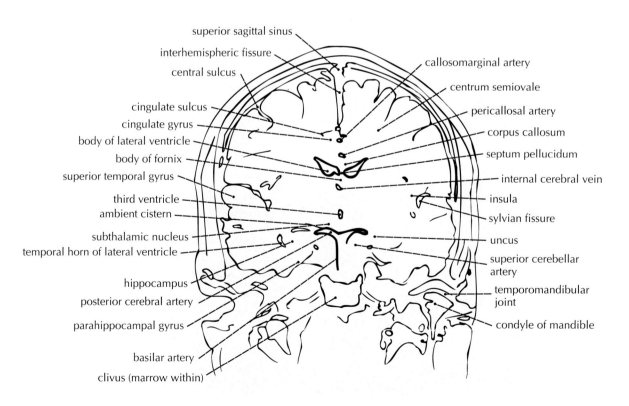

superior sagittal sinus

interhemispheric fissure

callosomarginal artery

central sulcus

centrum semiovale

cingulate sulcus

pericallosal artery

cingulate gyrus

corpus callosum

body of lateral ventricle

septum pellucidum

body of fornix

superior temporal gyrus

internal cerebral vein

third ventricle

insula

ambient cistern

sylvian fissure

subthalamic nucleus

uncus

temporal horn of lateral ventricle

superior cerebellar artery

hippocampus

temporomandibular joint

posterior cerebral artery

parahippocampal gyrus

condyle of mandible

basilar artery

clivus (marrow within)

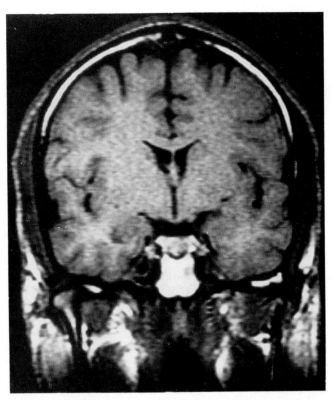

**2-38** Coronal MR scan through third ventricle (600/20).
Section 23 in Fig. 2-36.

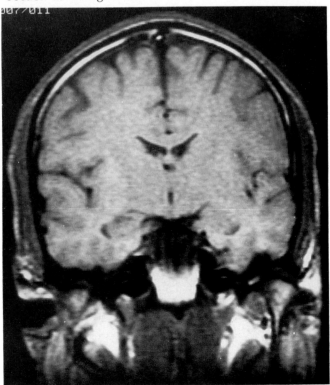

**2-39** Coronal MR scan through third ventricle and clivus
(600/20). Section 21 in Fig. 2-36.

# 2/Brain, Coronal MRI

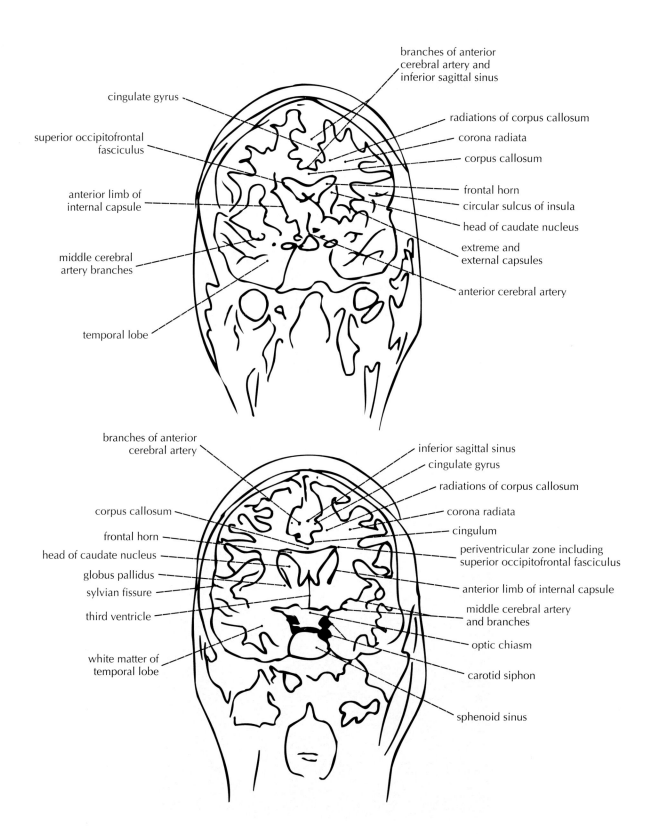

cingulate gyrus

superior occipitofrontal
fasciculus

anterior limb of
internal capsule

middle cerebral
artery branches

temporal lobe

branches of anterior
cerebral artery and
inferior sagittal sinus

radiations of corpus callosum

corona radiata

corpus callosum

frontal horn

circular sulcus of insula

head of caudate nucleus

extreme and
external capsules

anterior cerebral artery

branches of anterior
cerebral artery

corpus callosum

frontal horn

head of caudate nucleus

globus pallidus

sylvian fissure

third ventricle

white matter of
temporal lobe

inferior sagittal sinus

cingulate gyrus

radiations of corpus callosum

corona radiata

cingulum

periventricular zone including
superior occipitofrontal fasciculus

anterior limb of internal capsule

middle cerebral artery
and branches

optic chiasm

carotid siphon

sphenoid sinus

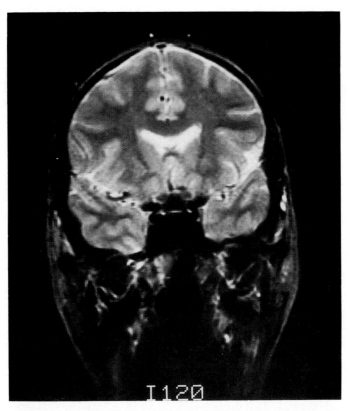

**2-40** Coronal MR scan through frontal horns (2000/90). Section 29 in Fig. 2-36.

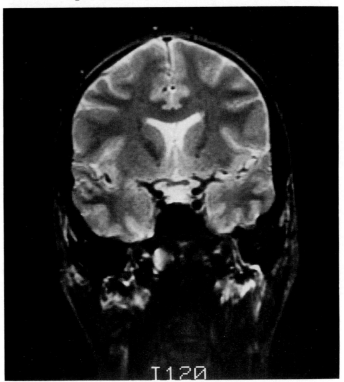

**2-41** Coronal MR scan through frontal horns (2000/90). Section 25 in Fig. 2-36.

# 2/Brain, Coronal MRI

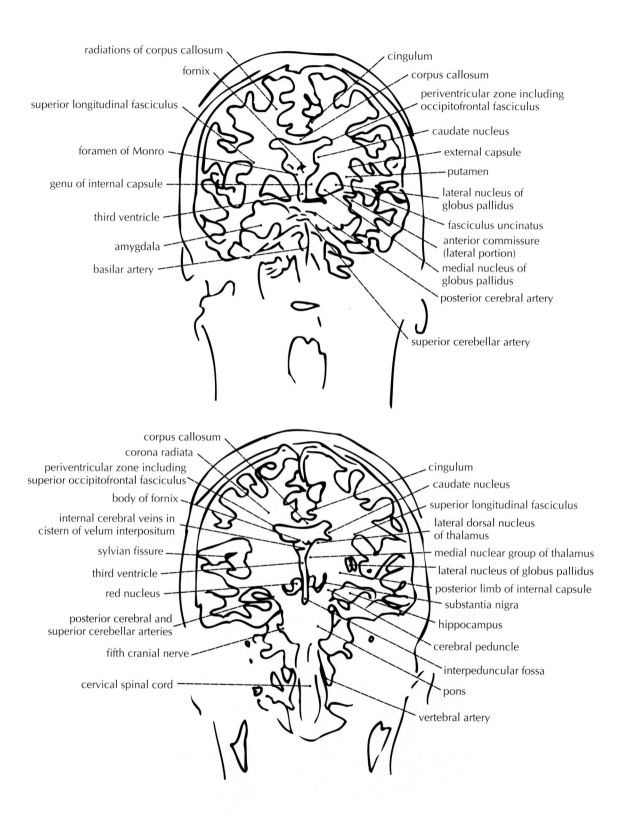

radiations of corpus callosum

cingulum

fornix

corpus callosum

superior longitudinal fasciculus

periventricular zone including
occipitofrontal fasciculus

caudate nucleus

foramen of Monro

external capsule

putamen

genu of internal capsule

lateral nucleus of
globus pallidus

third ventricle

fasciculus uncinatus

anterior commissure
(lateral portion)

amygdala

medial nucleus of
globus pallidus

basilar artery

posterior cerebral artery

superior cerebellar artery

corpus callosum

corona radiata

periventricular zone including
superior occipitofrontal fasciculus

cingulum

caudate nucleus

body of fornix

superior longitudinal fasciculus

internal cerebral veins in
cistern of velum interpositum

lateral dorsal nucleus
of thalamus

sylvian fissure

medial nuclear group of thalamus

third ventricle

lateral nucleus of globus pallidus

red nucleus

posterior limb of internal capsule

substantia nigra

posterior cerebral and
superior cerebellar arteries

hippocampus

fifth cranial nerve

cerebral peduncle

interpeduncular fossa

cervical spinal cord

pons

vertebral artery

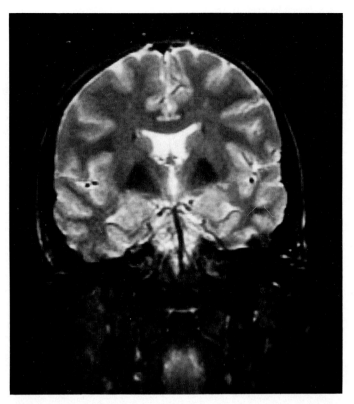

**2-42** Coronal MR scan through third ventricle and basal ganglia (2000/90). Section 21 in Fig. 2-36.

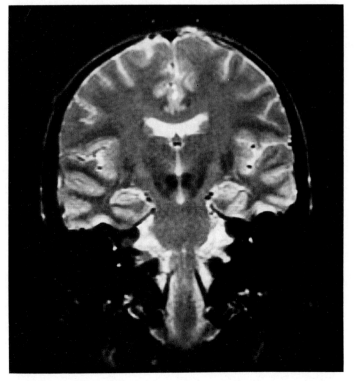

**2-43** Coronal MR scan through red nucleus (2000/90). Section 17 in Fig. 2-36.

# 2/Brain, Coronal MRI

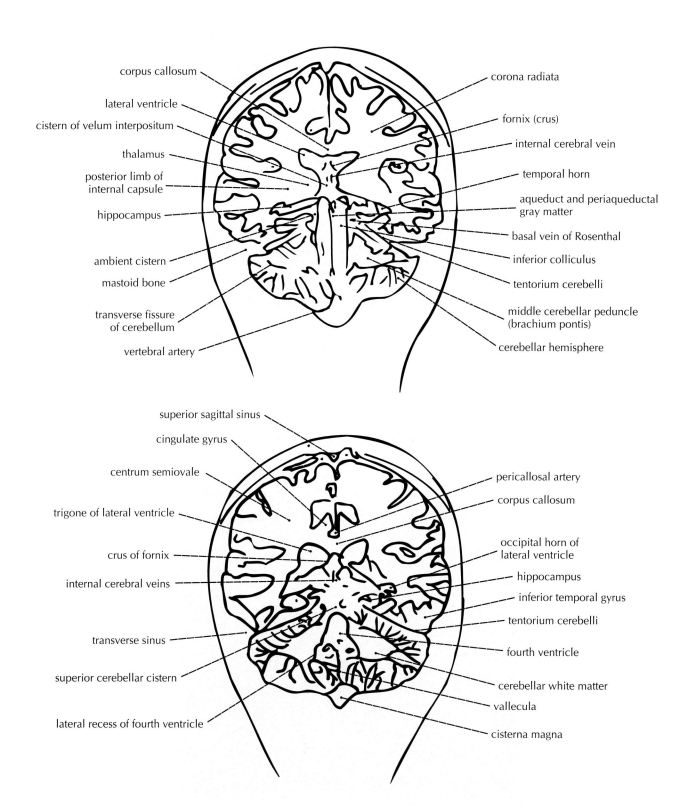

corpus callosum

lateral ventricle

cistern of velum interpositum

thalamus

posterior limb of
internal capsule

hippocampus

ambient cistern

mastoid bone

transverse fissure
of cerebellum

vertebral artery

corona radiata

fornix (crus)

internal cerebral vein

temporal horn

aqueduct and periaqueductal
gray matter

basal vein of Rosenthal

inferior colliculus

tentorium cerebelli

middle cerebellar peduncle
(brachium pontis)

cerebellar hemisphere

superior sagittal sinus

cingulate gyrus

centrum semiovale

trigone of lateral ventricle

crus of fornix

internal cerebral veins

transverse sinus

superior cerebellar cistern

lateral recess of fourth ventricle

pericallosal artery

corpus callosum

occipital horn of
lateral ventricle

hippocampus

inferior temporal gyrus

tentorium cerebelli

fourth ventricle

cerebellar white matter

vallecula

cisterna magna

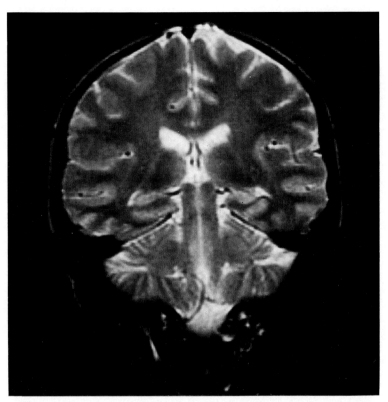

**2-44** Coronal MR scan through posterior body of corpus callosum (2000/90). Section 15 in Fig. 2-36.

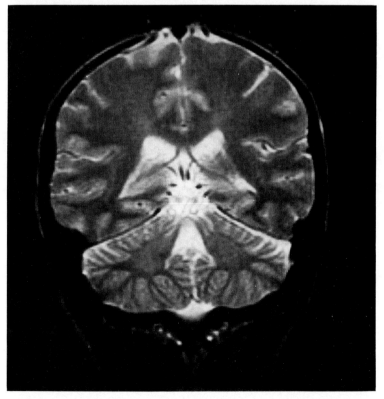

**2-45** Coronal MR scan through fourth ventricle (2000/90). Section 13 in Fig. 2-36.

# 2/Brain, Coronal MRI

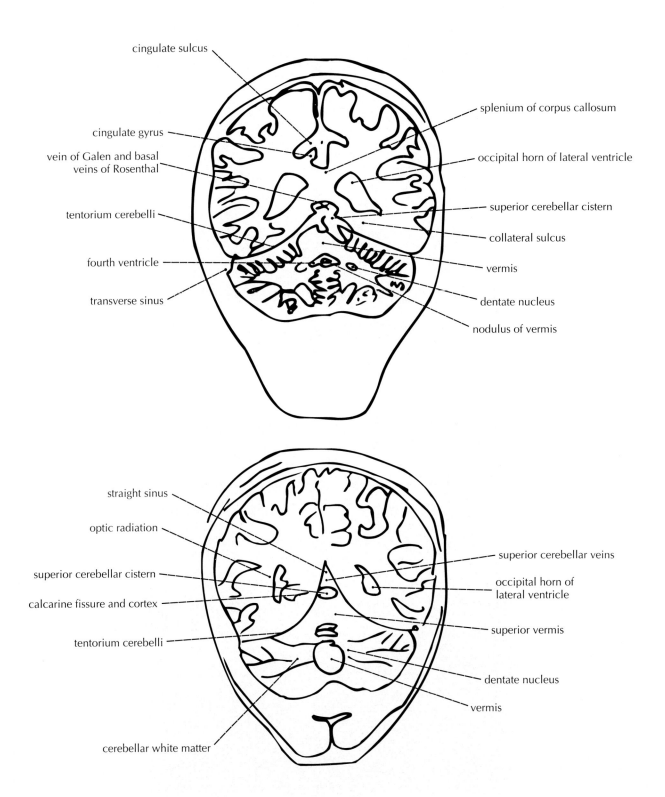

cingulate sulcus

splenium of corpus callosum

cingulate gyrus

vein of Galen and basal
veins of Rosenthal

occipital horn of lateral ventricle

tentorium cerebelli

superior cerebellar cistern

collateral sulcus

fourth ventricle

vermis

transverse sinus

dentate nucleus

nodulus of vermis

straight sinus

optic radiation

superior cerebellar veins

superior cerebellar cistern

occipital horn of
lateral ventricle

calcarine fissure and cortex

tentorium cerebelli

superior vermis

dentate nucleus

vermis

cerebellar white matter

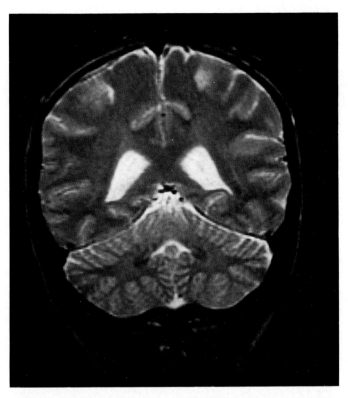

**2-46** Coronal MR scan through fourth ventricle (2000/90). Section 11 in Fig. 2-36.

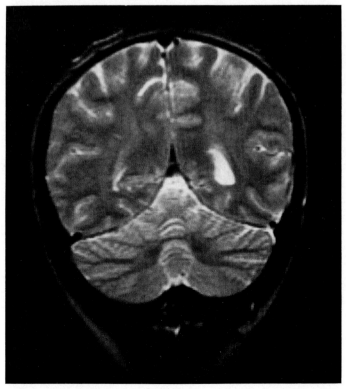

**2-47** Coronal MR scan through posterior fossa (2000/90). Section 5 in Fig. 2-36.

# 2/Brain, Coronal MRI

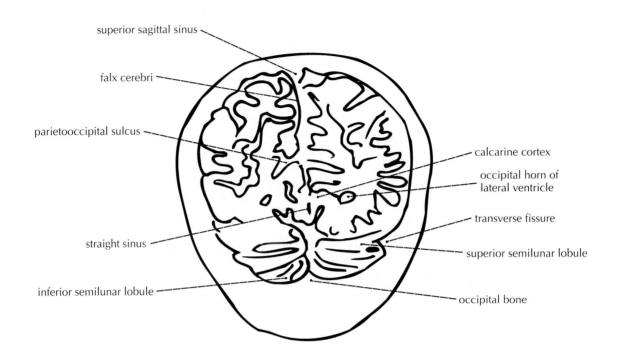

superior sagittal sinus

falx cerebri

parietooccipital sulcus

calcarine cortex

occipital horn of lateral ventricle

transverse fissure

straight sinus

superior semilunar lobule

inferior semilunar lobule

occipital bone

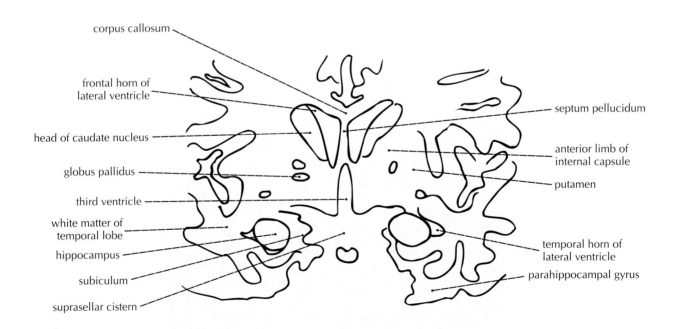

corpus callosum

frontal horn of lateral ventricle

septum pellucidum

head of caudate nucleus

anterior limb of internal capsule

globus pallidus

putamen

third ventricle

white matter of temporal lobe

hippocampus

temporal horn of lateral ventricle

subiculum

parahippocampal gyrus

suprasellar cistern

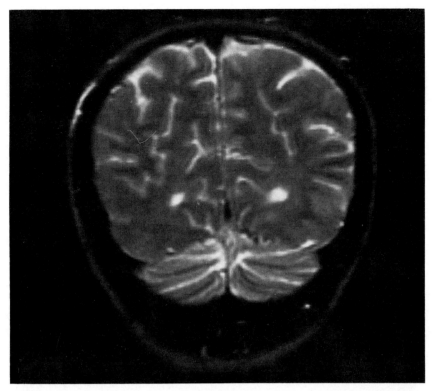

**2-48** Coronal MR scan through posterior fossa (2000/90). Section 3 in Fig. 2-36.

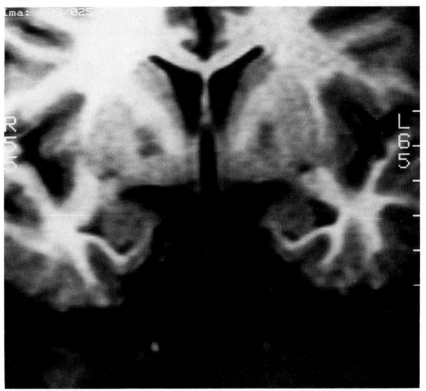

**2-49** Coronal MR scan through basal ganglia (150/10, flip angle 60°). Magnified section through level 27 in Fig. 2-36.

# 2/Brain, Axial Scout and Sagittal MRI

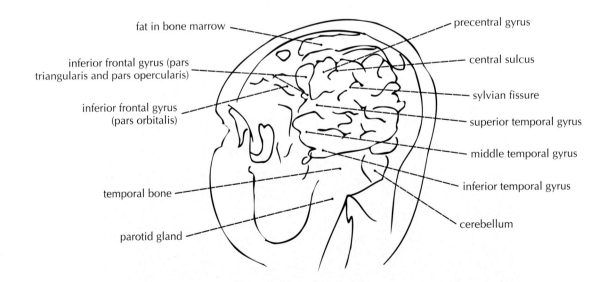

fat in bone marrow

inferior frontal gyrus (pars triangularis and pars opercularis)

inferior frontal gyrus (pars orbitalis)

temporal bone

parotid gland

precentral gyrus

central sulcus

sylvian fissure

superior temporal gyrus

middle temporal gyrus

inferior temporal gyrus

cerebellum

# 2/Brain, Axial Scout and Sagittal MRI

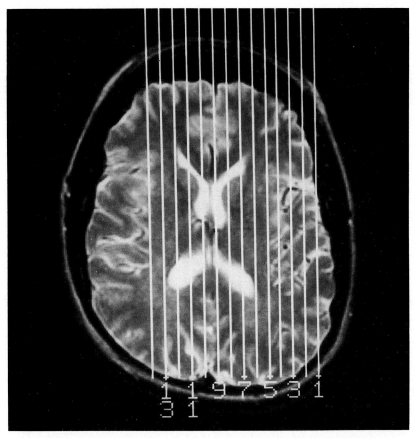

**2-50** This axial scout MR scan is used to illustrate the locations of sagittal MR sections. Sections 1, 2, 3, 5, 6, 7, 8, and 9 will be shown.

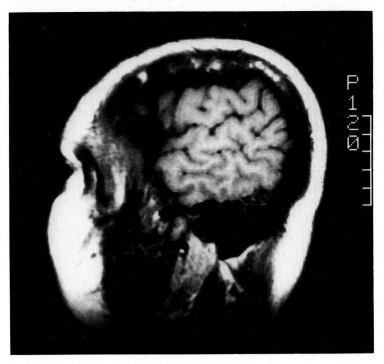

**2-51** Sagittal MR scan through temporal lobe (600/15). Section 1 in Fig. 2-50.

# 2/Brain, Sagittal MRI

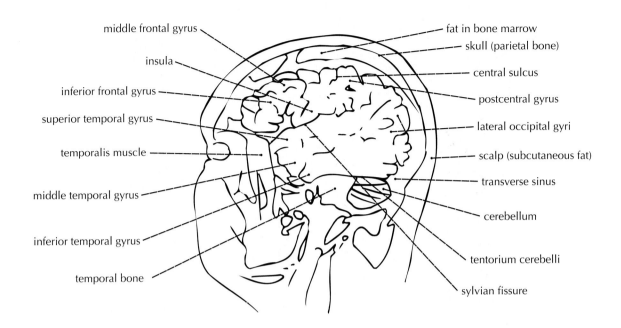

middle frontal gyrus

insula

inferior frontal gyrus

superior temporal gyrus

temporalis muscle

middle temporal gyrus

inferior temporal gyrus

temporal bone

fat in bone marrow

skull (parietal bone)

central sulcus

postcentral gyrus

lateral occipital gyri

scalp (subcutaneous fat)

transverse sinus

cerebellum

tentorium cerebelli

sylvian fissure

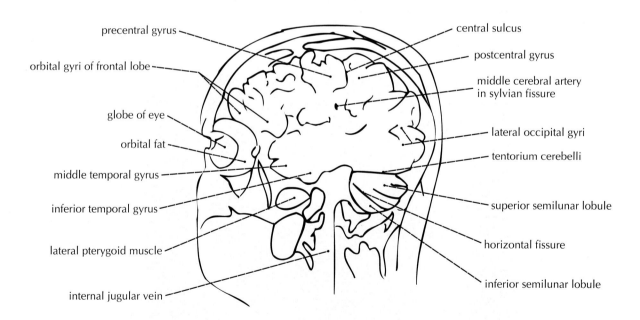

precentral gyrus

orbital gyri of frontal lobe

globe of eye

orbital fat

middle temporal gyrus

inferior temporal gyrus

lateral pterygoid muscle

internal jugular vein

central sulcus

postcentral gyrus

middle cerebral artery
in sylvian fissure

lateral occipital gyri

tentorium cerebelli

superior semilunar lobule

horizontal fissure

inferior semilunar lobule

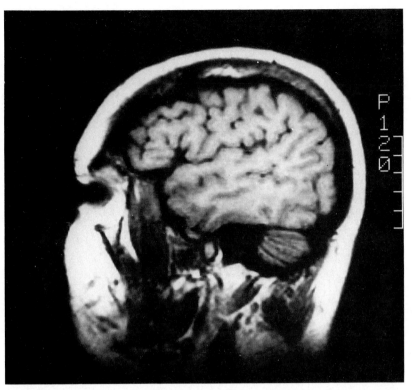

**2-52** Sagittal MR scan through temporal lobe (600/15). Section 2 in Fig. 2-50.

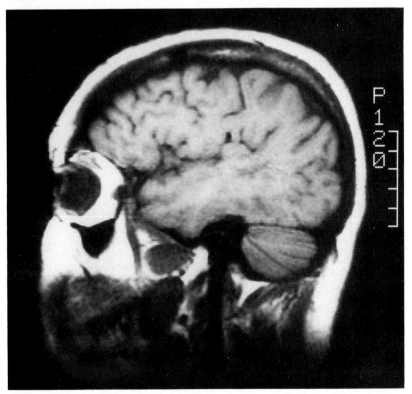

**2-53** Sagittal MR scan through temporal lobe (600/15). Section 3 in Fig. 2-50.

# 2/Brain, Sagittal MRI

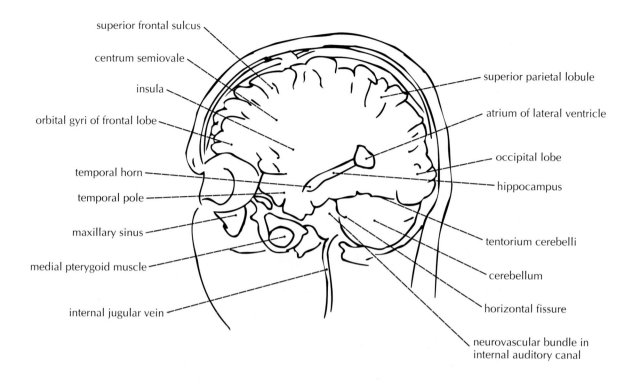

superior frontal sulcus

centrum semiovale

insula

orbital gyri of frontal lobe

temporal horn

temporal pole

maxillary sinus

medial pterygoid muscle

internal jugular vein

superior parietal lobule

atrium of lateral ventricle

occipital lobe

hippocampus

tentorium cerebelli

cerebellum

horizontal fissure

neurovascular bundle in
internal auditory canal

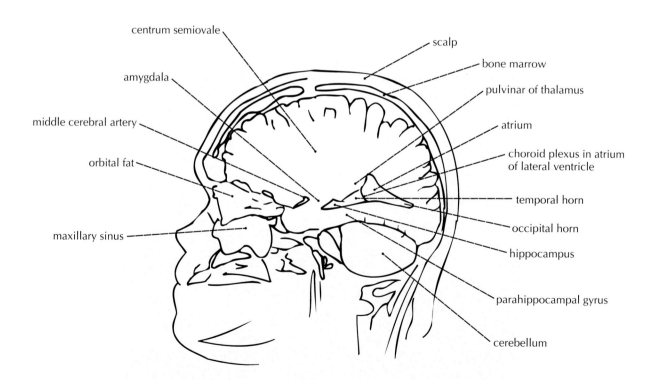

centrum semiovale

amygdala

middle cerebral artery

orbital fat

maxillary sinus

scalp

bone marrow

pulvinar of thalamus

atrium

choroid plexus in atrium
of lateral ventricle

temporal horn

occipital horn

hippocampus

parahippocampal gyrus

cerebellum

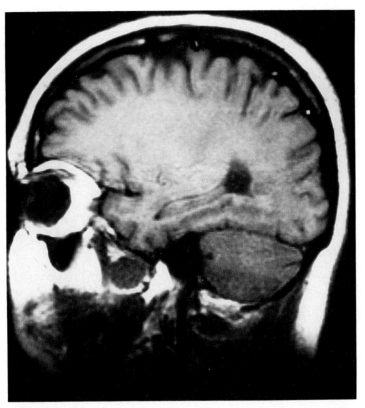

**2-54** Sagittal MR scan through atrium and temporal horn (600/15). Section 5 in Fig. 2-50.

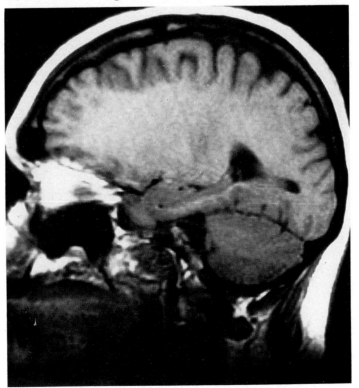

**2-55** Sagittal MR scan through occipital horn (600/15). Section 6 in Fig. 2-50.

# 2/Brain, Sagittal MRI

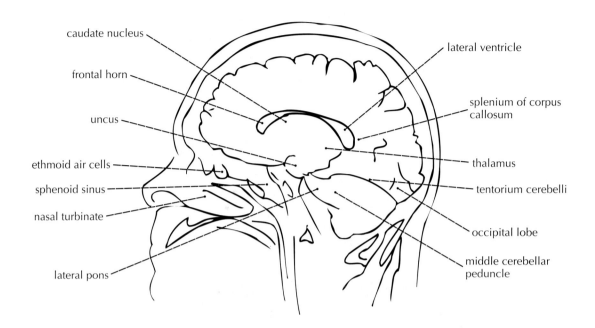

caudate nucleus

frontal horn

uncus

ethmoid air cells

sphenoid sinus

nasal turbinate

lateral pons

lateral ventricle

splenium of corpus callosum

thalamus

tentorium cerebelli

occipital lobe

middle cerebellar peduncle

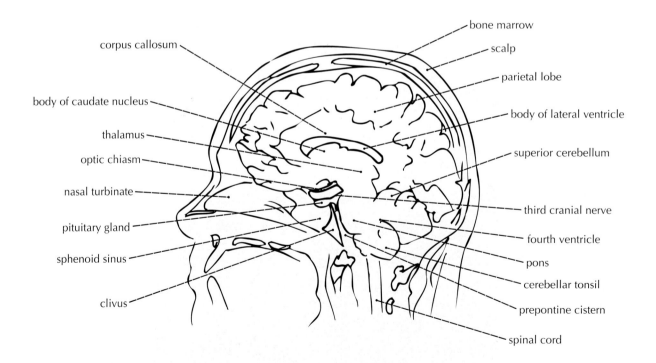

corpus callosum

body of caudate nucleus

thalamus

optic chiasm

nasal turbinate

pituitary gland

sphenoid sinus

clivus

bone marrow

scalp

parietal lobe

body of lateral ventricle

superior cerebellum

third cranial nerve

fourth ventricle

pons

cerebellar tonsil

prepontine cistern

spinal cord

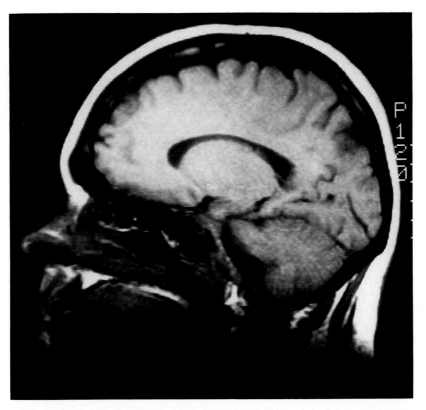

**2-56** Sagittal MR scan through lateral ventricle and thalamus (600/15).
Section 7 in Fig. 2-50.

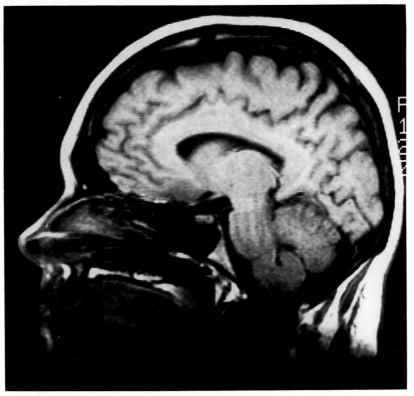

**2-57** Sagittal MR scan through lateral ventricle and thalamus (600/15).
Section 8 in Fig. 2-50.

# 2/Brain, Sagittal MRI

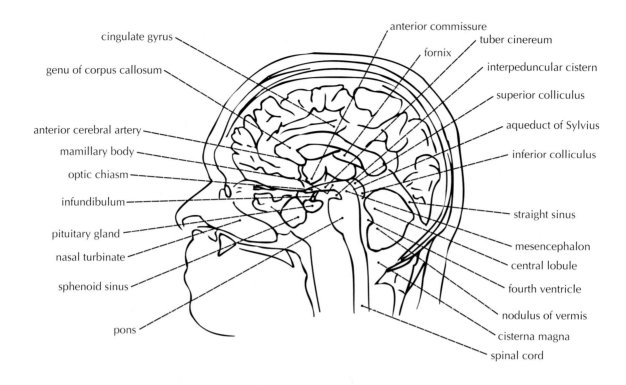

cingulate gyrus

genu of corpus callosum

anterior cerebral artery

mamillary body

optic chiasm

infundibulum

pituitary gland

nasal turbinate

sphenoid sinus

pons

anterior commissure

fornix

tuber cinereum

interpeduncular cistern

superior colliculus

aqueduct of Sylvius

inferior colliculus

straight sinus

mesencephalon

central lobule

fourth ventricle

nodulus of vermis

cisterna magna

spinal cord

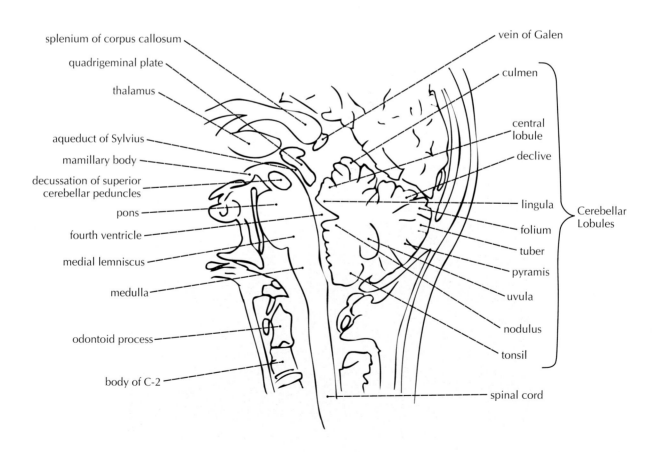

splenium of corpus callosum

quadrigeminal plate

thalamus

aqueduct of Sylvius

mamillary body

decussation of superior
cerebellar peduncles

pons

fourth ventricle

medial lemniscus

medulla

odontoid process

body of C-2

vein of Galen

culmen

central
lobule

declive

lingula

folium

tuber

pyramis

uvula

nodulus

tonsil

Cerebellar
Lobules

spinal cord

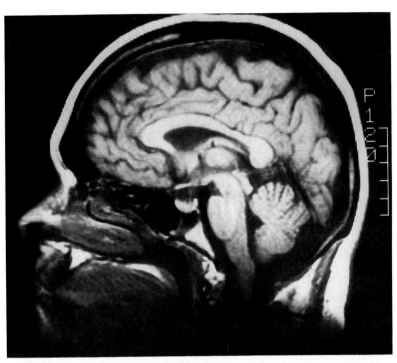

**2-58** Sagittal MR scan of the midline (600/15). Section 9 in Fig. 2-50.

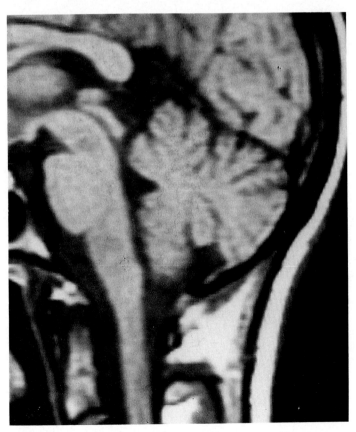

**2-59** Sagittal MR scan through cerebellum, midline section (600/15).

# 2/Brain, Sagittal Scout MRI and Axial MRI (Infant)

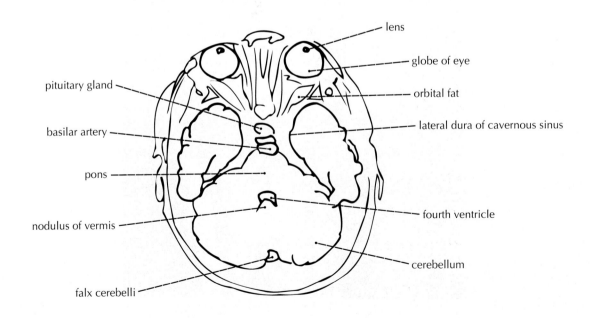

lens

globe of eye

orbital fat

pituitary gland

lateral dura of cavernous sinus

basilar artery

pons

fourth ventricle

nodulus of vermis

cerebellum

falx cerebelli

# 2/Brain, Sagittal Scout MRI and Axial MRI (Infant)

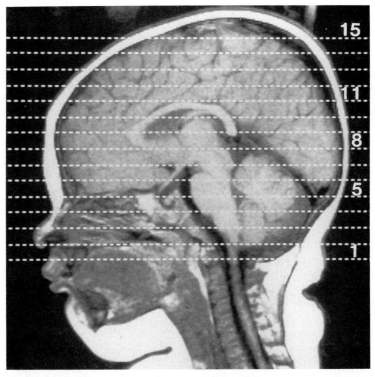

**2-60** Sagittal scout MR scan for demonstration of the axial MR sections. Sections 5, 8, and 11 will be shown.

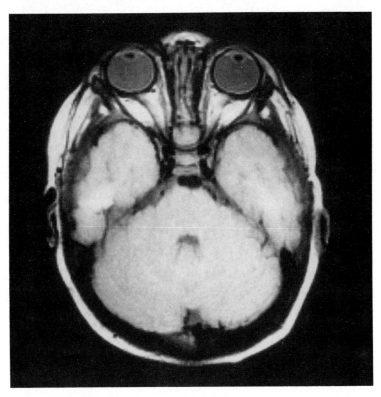

**2-61** Axial MR scan of a 5-month-old infant (2000/30). Section 5 in Fig. 2-60.

# 2/Brain, Axial MRI (Infant)

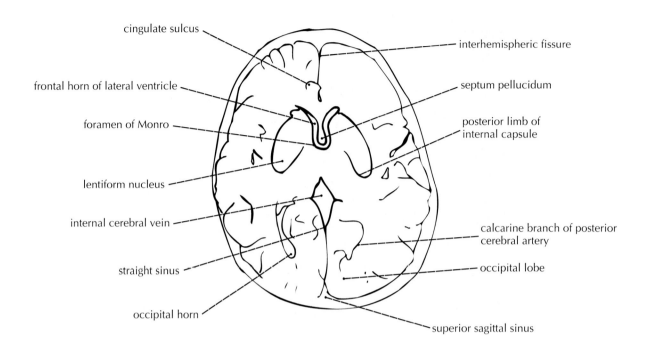

cingulate sulcus

interhemispheric fissure

frontal horn of lateral ventricle

septum pellucidum

foramen of Monro

posterior limb of internal capsule

lentiform nucleus

internal cerebral vein

calcarine branch of posterior cerebral artery

straight sinus

occipital lobe

occipital horn

superior sagittal sinus

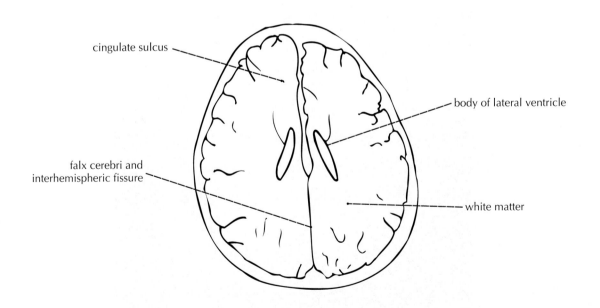

cingulate sulcus

body of lateral ventricle

falx cerebri and interhemispheric fissure

white matter

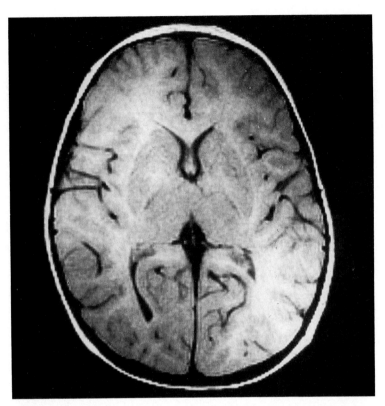

**2-62** Axial MR scan of a 5-month-old infant (2000/30). Section 8 in Fig. 2-60.

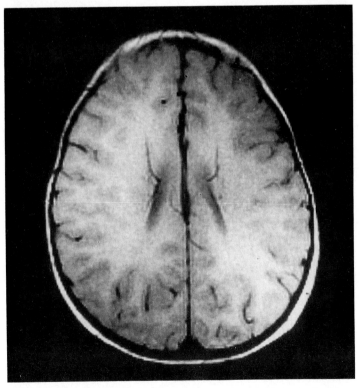

**2-63** Axial MR scan of a 5-month-old infant (2000/30). Section 11 in Fig. 2-60.

# 2/Brain, Axial MRI (Infant)

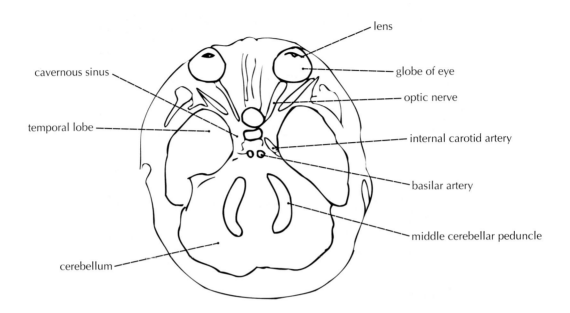

lens

globe of eye

optic nerve

cavernous sinus

internal carotid artery

temporal lobe

basilar artery

middle cerebellar peduncle

cerebellum

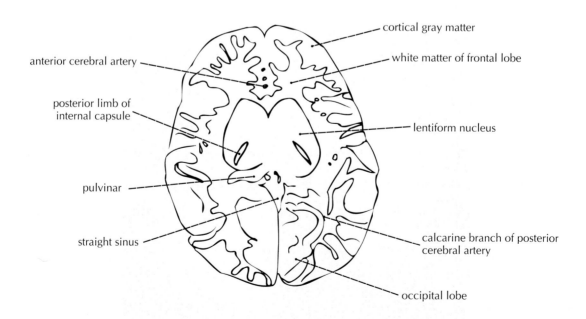

cortical gray matter

white matter of frontal lobe

anterior cerebral artery

posterior limb of
internal capsule

lentiform nucleus

pulvinar

straight sinus

calcarine branch of posterior
cerebral artery

occipital lobe

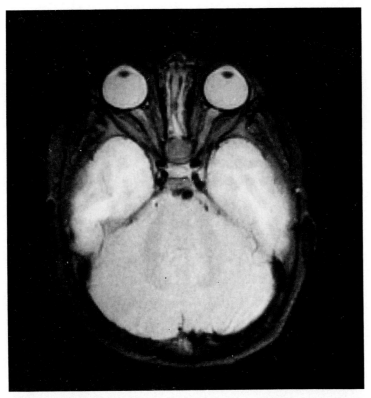

**2-64** Axial MR scan of a 5-month-old infant (2000/60). Section 5 in Fig. 2-60.

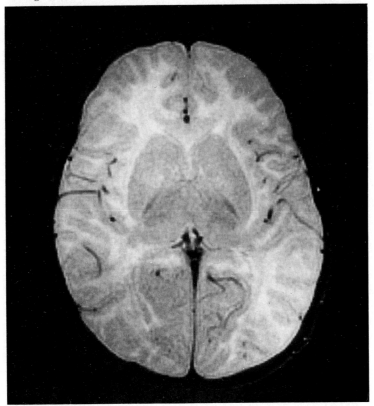

**2-65** Axial MR scan of a 5-month-old infant (2000/60). Section 8 in Fig. 2-60.

# 2/Brain, Axial MRI (Infant)

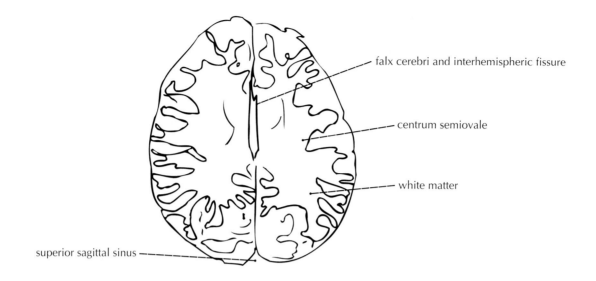

falx cerebri and interhemispheric fissure

centrum semiovale

white matter

superior sagittal sinus

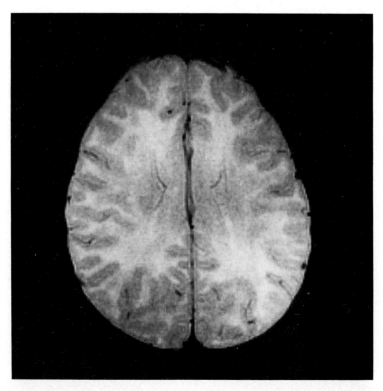

**2-66** Axial MR scan of a 5-month-old infant (2000/60). Section 11 in Fig. 2-60.

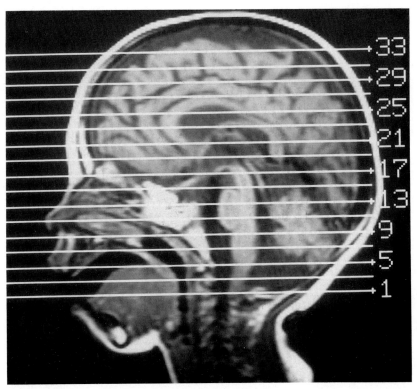

**2-67** Sagittal scout MR scan for demonstration of axial MR sections. Sections 9, 15, 19, 21, and 25 will be shown.

# 2/Brain, Axial MRI (Infant)

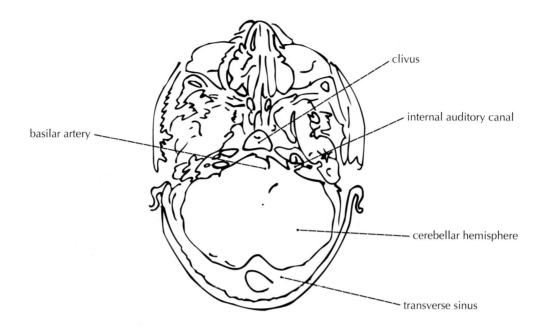

clivus

internal auditory canal

basilar artery

cerebellar hemisphere

transverse sinus

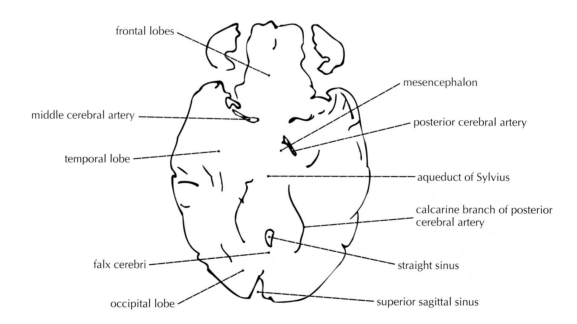

frontal lobes

mesencephalon

middle cerebral artery

posterior cerebral artery

temporal lobe

aqueduct of Sylvius

calcarine branch of posterior cerebral artery

falx cerebri

straight sinus

occipital lobe

superior sagittal sinus

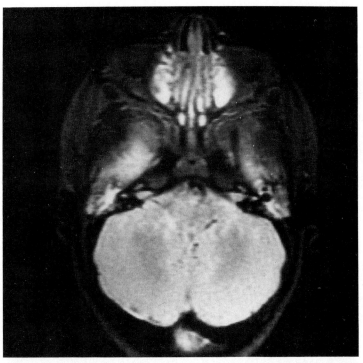

**2-68** Axial MR scan of a 9-month-old infant (2000/80). Section 9 in Fig. 2-67.

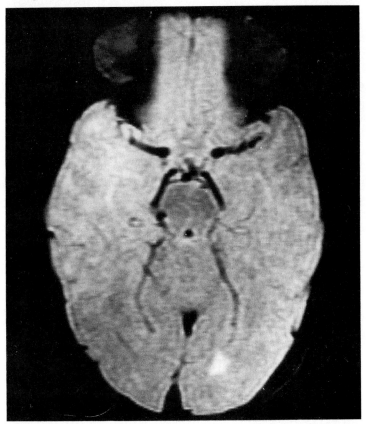

**2-69** Axial MR scan of a 9-month-old infant (2000/80). Section 15 in Fig. 2-67.

# 2/Brain, Axial MRI (Infant)

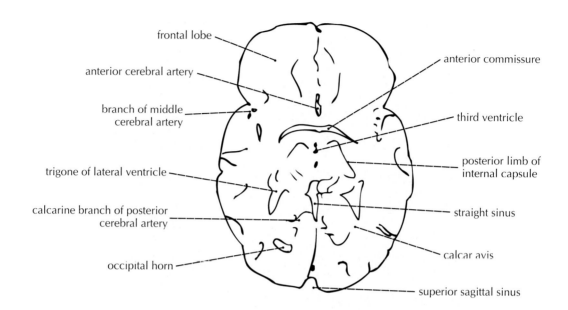

frontal lobe

anterior cerebral artery

branch of middle
cerebral artery

trigone of lateral ventricle

calcarine branch of posterior
cerebral artery

occipital horn

anterior commissure

third ventricle

posterior limb of
internal capsule

straight sinus

calcar avis

superior sagittal sinus

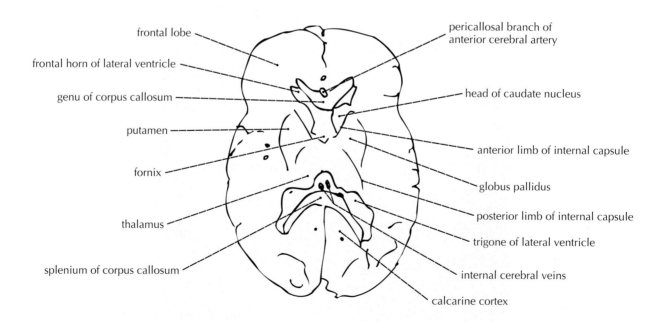

frontal lobe

frontal horn of lateral ventricle

genu of corpus callosum

putamen

fornix

thalamus

splenium of corpus callosum

pericallosal branch of
anterior cerebral artery

head of caudate nucleus

anterior limb of internal capsule

globus pallidus

posterior limb of internal capsule

trigone of lateral ventricle

internal cerebral veins

calcarine cortex

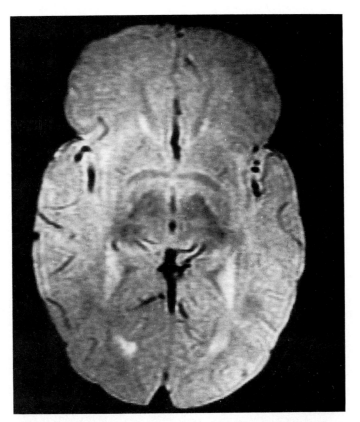

**2-70** Axial MR scan of a 9-month-old infant (2000/80). Section 19 in Fig. 2-67.

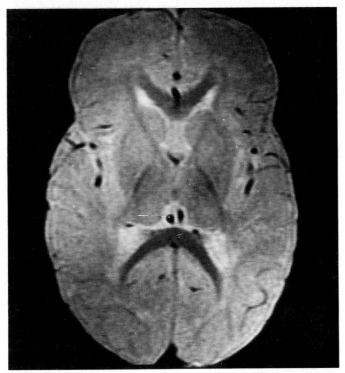

**2-71** Axial MR scan of a 9-month-old infant (2000/80). Section 21 in Fig. 2-67.

# 2/Brain, Axial MRI (Infant)

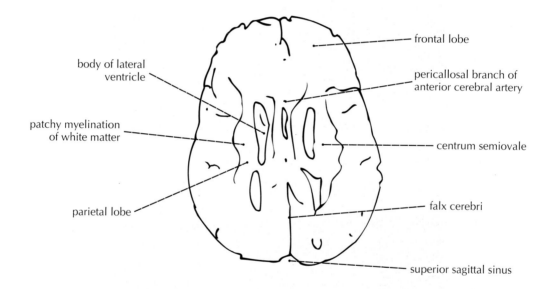

body of lateral
ventricle

patchy myelination
of white matter

parietal lobe

frontal lobe

pericallosal branch of
anterior cerebral artery

centrum semiovale

falx cerebri

superior sagittal sinus

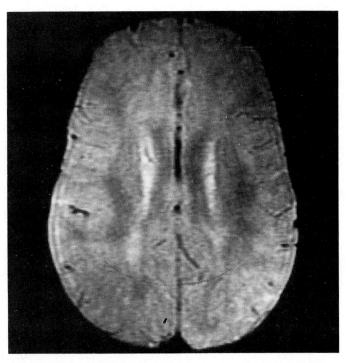

**2-72** Axial MR scan of a 9-month-old infant (2000/80). Section 25 in Fig. 2-67.

# 2/Head, Angiography

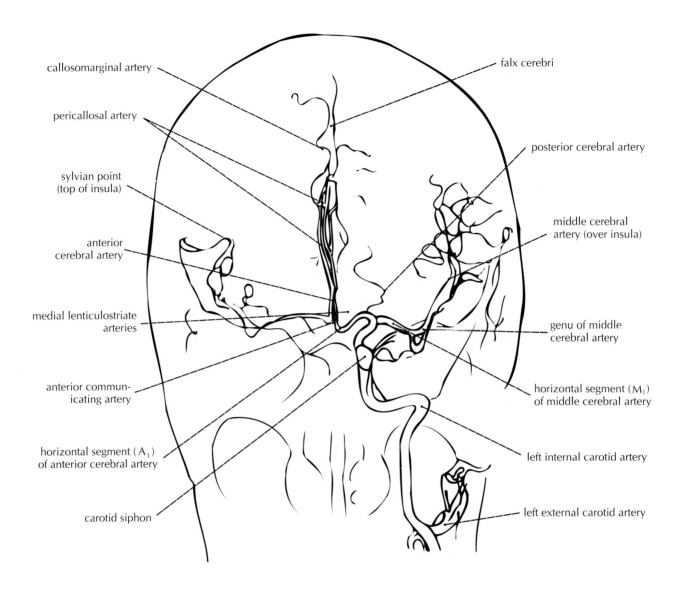

callosomarginal artery

pericallosal artery

sylvian point
(top of insula)

anterior
cerebral artery

medial lenticulostriate
arteries

anterior commun-
icating artery

horizontal segment (A$_1$)
of anterior cerebral artery

carotid siphon

falx cerebri

posterior cerebral artery

middle cerebral
artery (over insula)

genu of middle
cerebral artery

horizontal segment (M$_1$)
of middle cerebral artery

left internal carotid artery

left external carotid artery

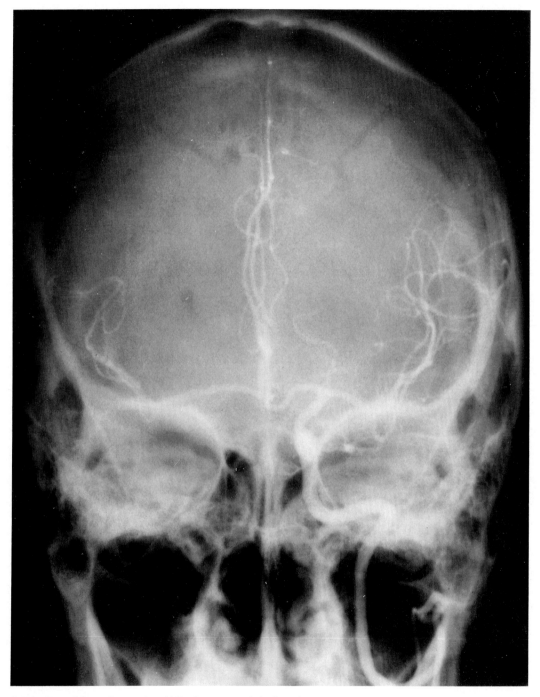

**2-73** Carotid angiography (AP view, arterial phase).

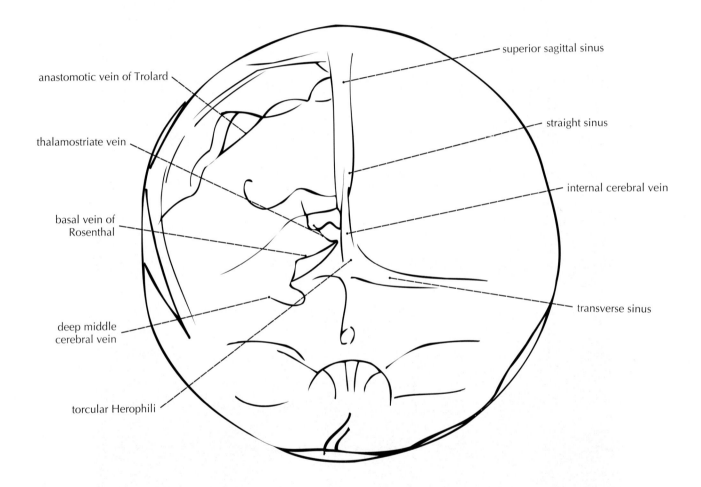

anastomotic vein of Trolard

thalamostriate vein

basal vein of
Rosenthal

deep middle
cerebral vein

torcular Herophili

superior sagittal sinus

straight sinus

internal cerebral vein

transverse sinus

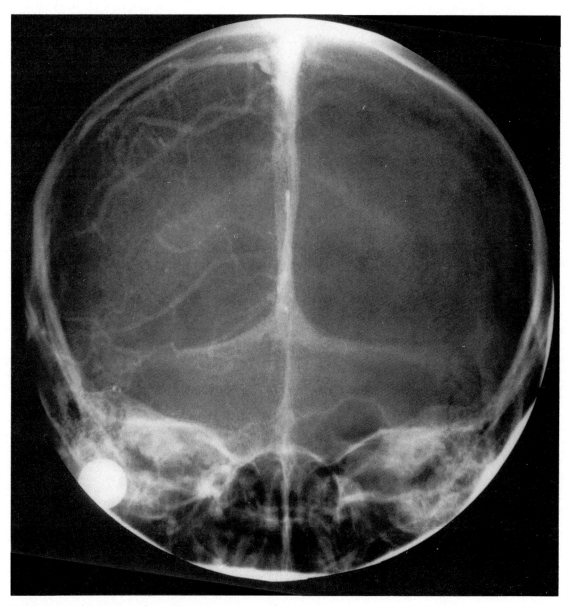

**2-74** Carotid angiography (AP view, venous phase).

# 2/Head, Angiography

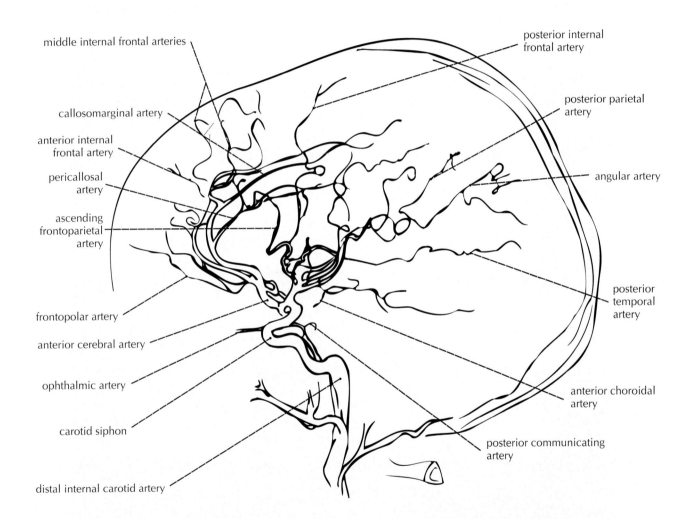

middle internal frontal arteries

posterior internal
frontal artery

posterior parietal
artery

callosomarginal artery

anterior internal
frontal artery

angular artery

pericallosal
artery

ascending
frontoparietal
artery

posterior
temporal
artery

frontopolar artery

anterior cerebral artery

ophthalmic artery

anterior choroidal
artery

carotid siphon

posterior communicating
artery

distal internal carotid artery

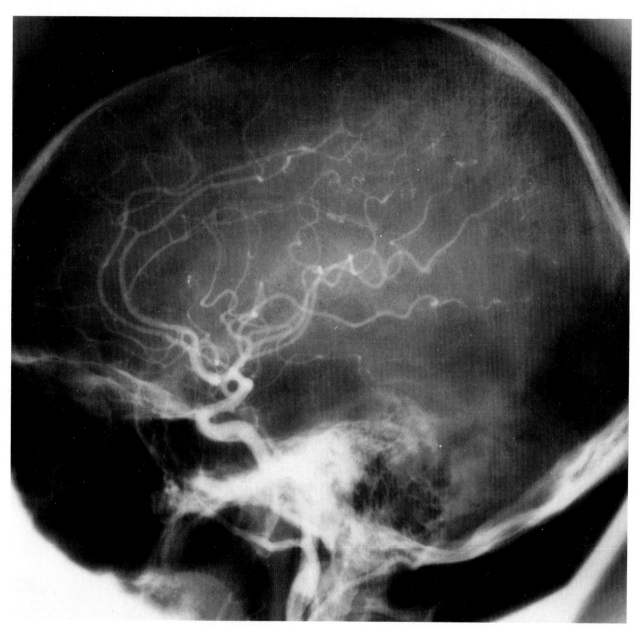

**2-75** Carotid angiography (lateral view, arterial phase).

# 2/Head, Angiography

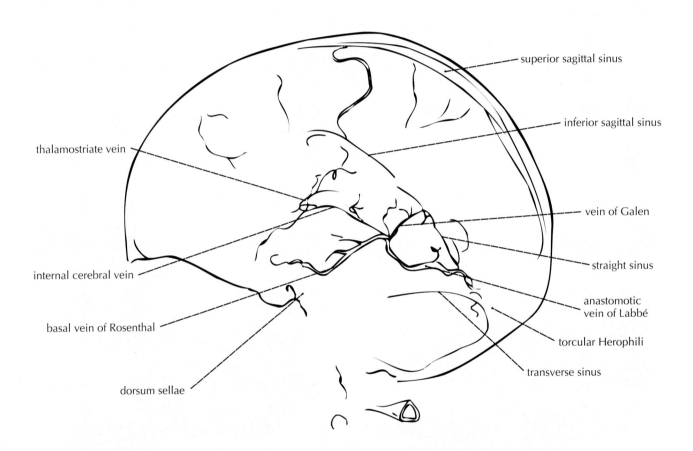

thalamostriate vein

internal cerebral vein

basal vein of Rosenthal

dorsum sellae

superior sagittal sinus

inferior sagittal sinus

vein of Galen

straight sinus

anastomotic
vein of Labbé

torcular Herophili

transverse sinus

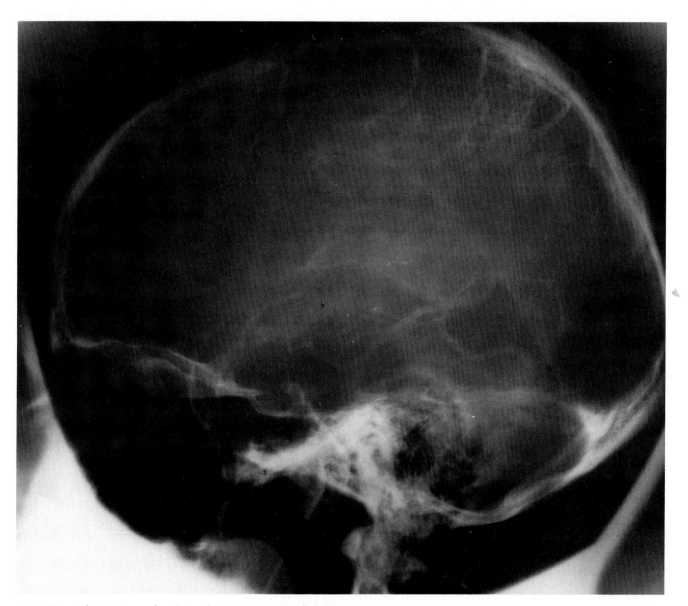

**2-76** Carotid arteriography (lateral view, venous phase).

# 2/Head, Angiography

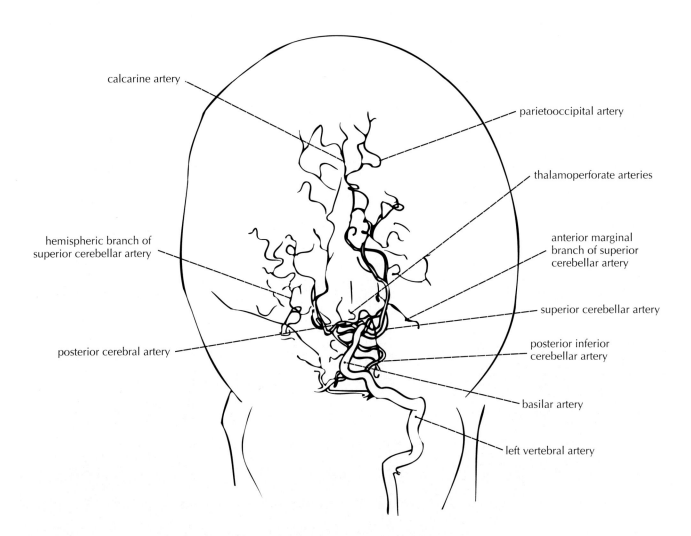

calcarine artery

parietooccipital artery

thalamoperforate arteries

hemispheric branch of
superior cerebellar artery

anterior marginal
branch of superior
cerebellar artery

superior cerebellar artery

posterior cerebral artery

posterior inferior
cerebellar artery

basilar artery

left vertebral artery

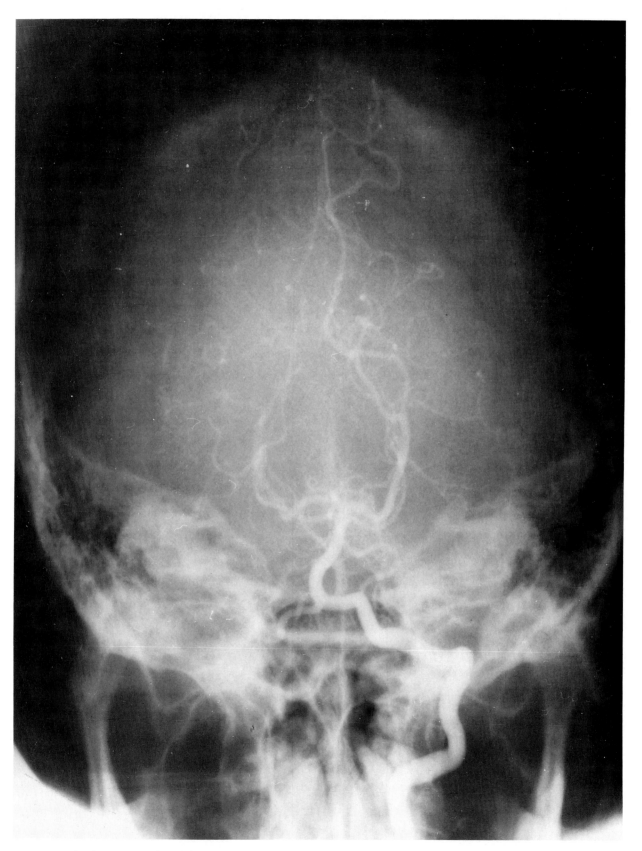

**2-77** Vertebral angiography (AP view, arterial phase).

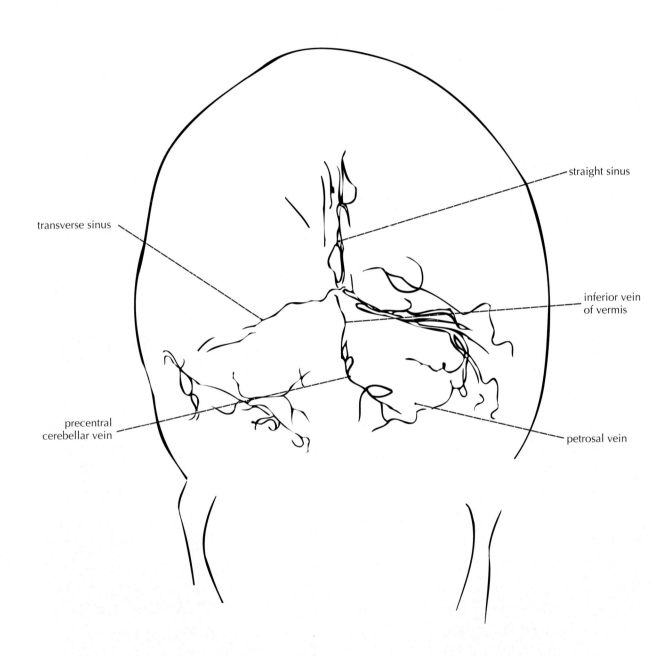

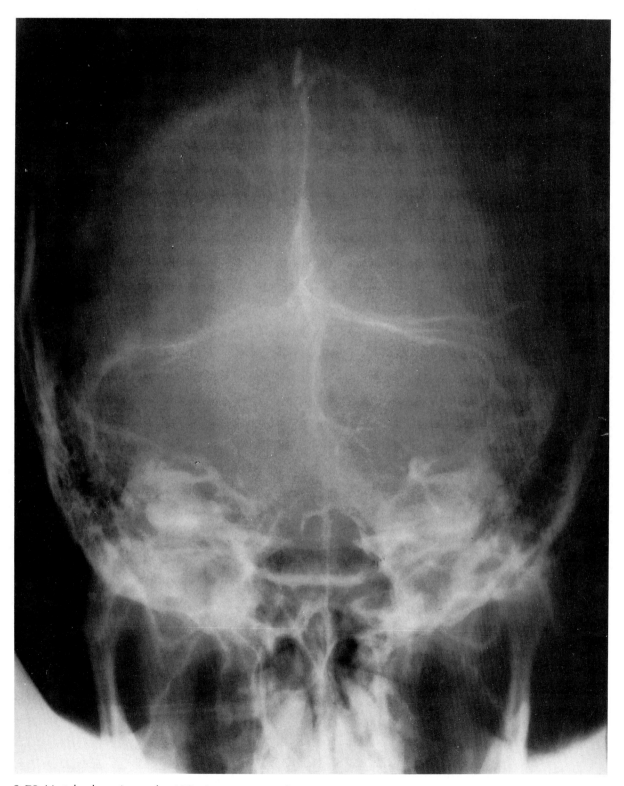

**2-78** Vertebral angiography (AP view, venous phase).

# 2/Head, Angiography

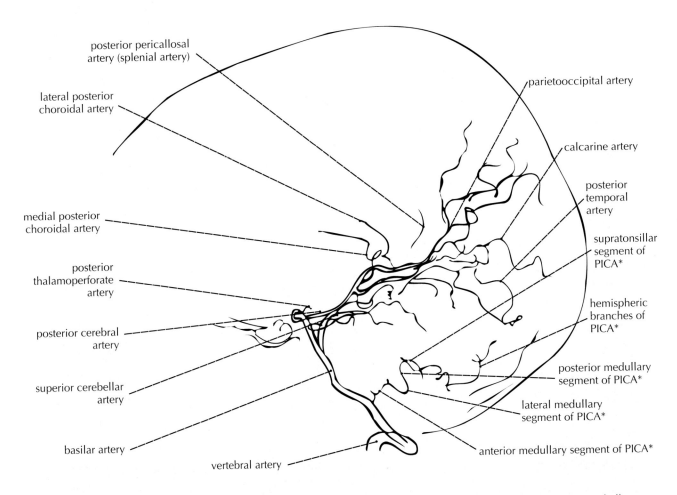

posterior pericallosal
artery (splenial artery)

lateral posterior
choroidal artery

medial posterior
choroidal artery

posterior
thalamoperforate
artery

posterior cerebral
artery

superior cerebellar
artery

basilar artery

vertebral artery

parietooccipital artery

calcarine artery

posterior
temporal
artery

supratonsillar
segment of
PICA*

hemispheric
branches of
PICA*

posterior medullary
segment of PICA*

lateral medullary
segment of PICA*

anterior medullary segment of PICA*

*PICA = posterior inferior cerebellar artery

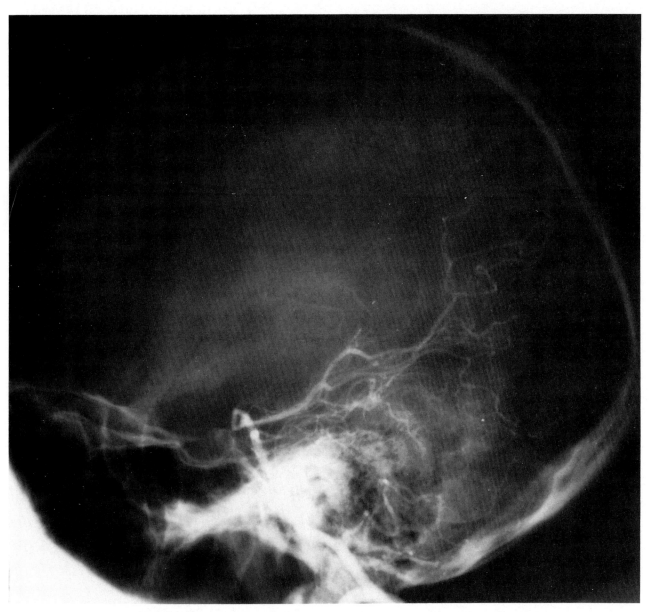

**2-79** Vertebral angiography (lateral view, arterial phase).

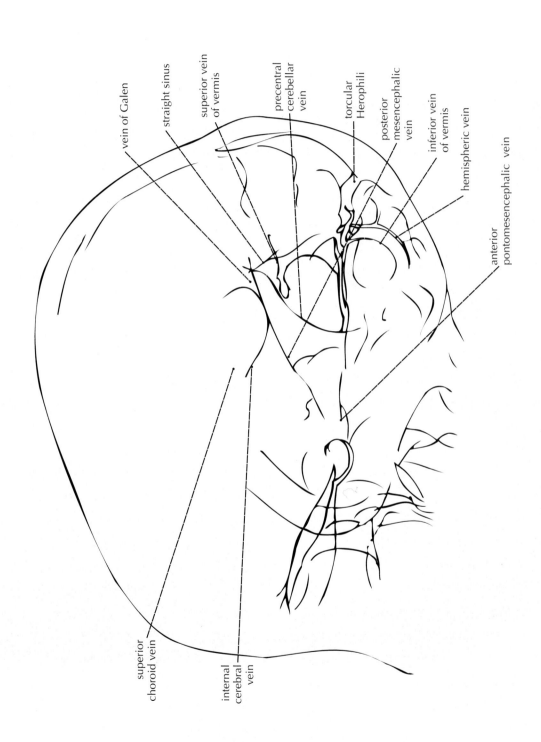

vein of Galen

straight sinus

superior vein of vermis

precentral cerebellar vein

torcular Herophili

posterior mesencephalic vein

inferior vein of vermis

hemispheric vein

anterior pontomesencephalic vein

superior choroid vein

internal cerebral vein

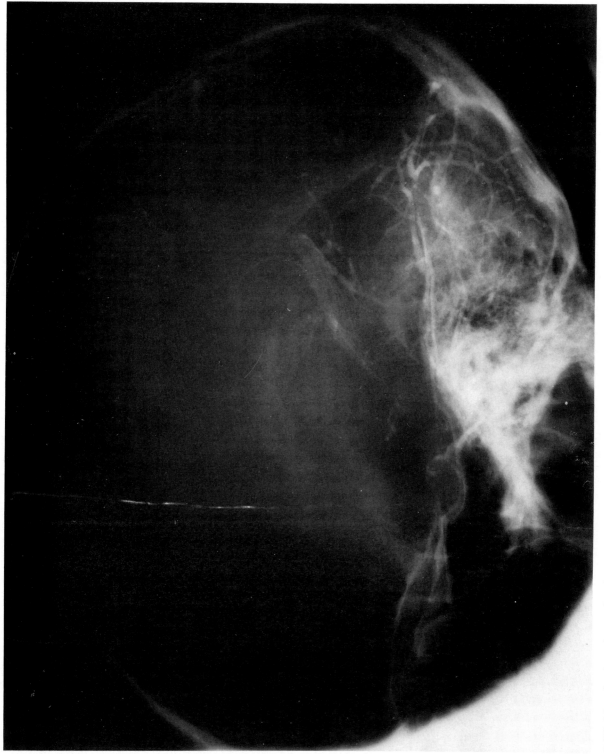

**2-80** Vertebral angiography (lateral view, venous phase).

# 2/Head, MR Angiography

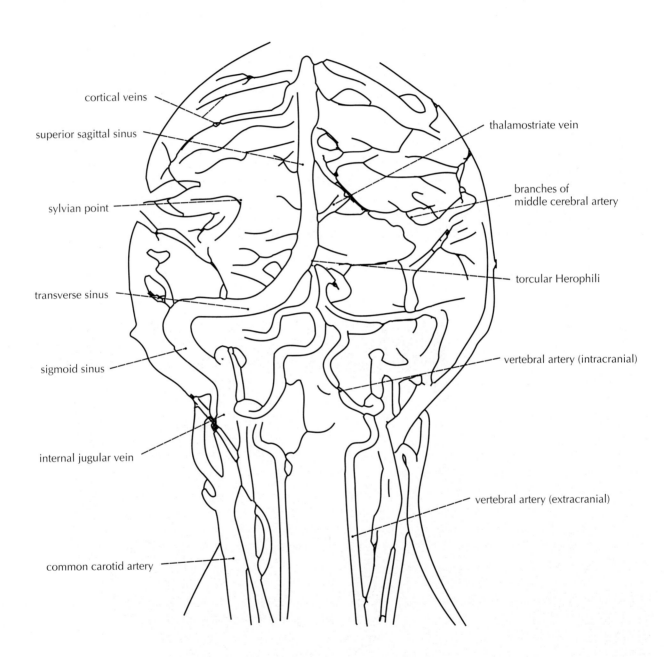

cortical veins

superior sagittal sinus

sylvian point

transverse sinus

sigmoid sinus

internal jugular vein

common carotid artery

thalamostriate vein

branches of
middle cerebral artery

torcular Herophili

vertebral artery (intracranial)

vertebral artery (extracranial)

# 2/Head, MR Angiography

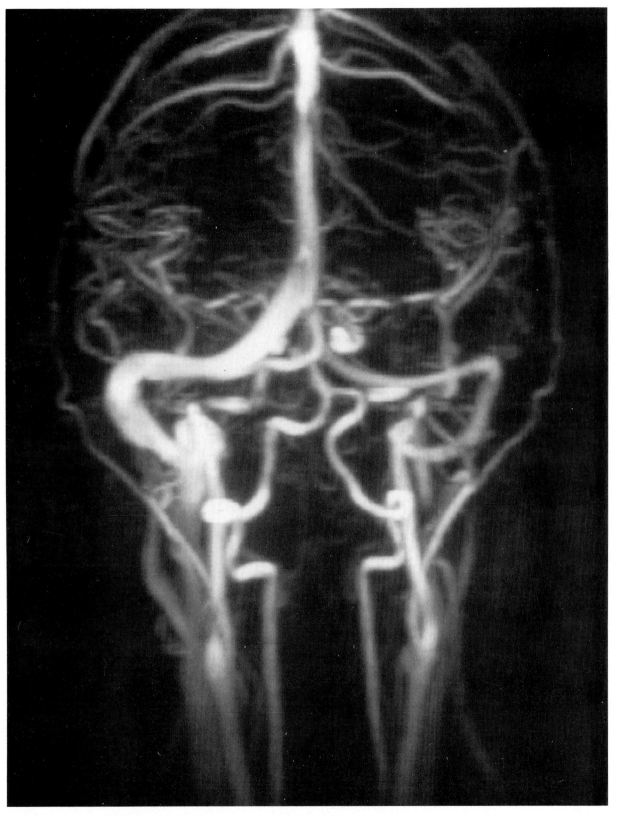

**2-81** Intracranial angiography (noncontrast MR scan, frontal view).

# 2/Head, MR Angiography

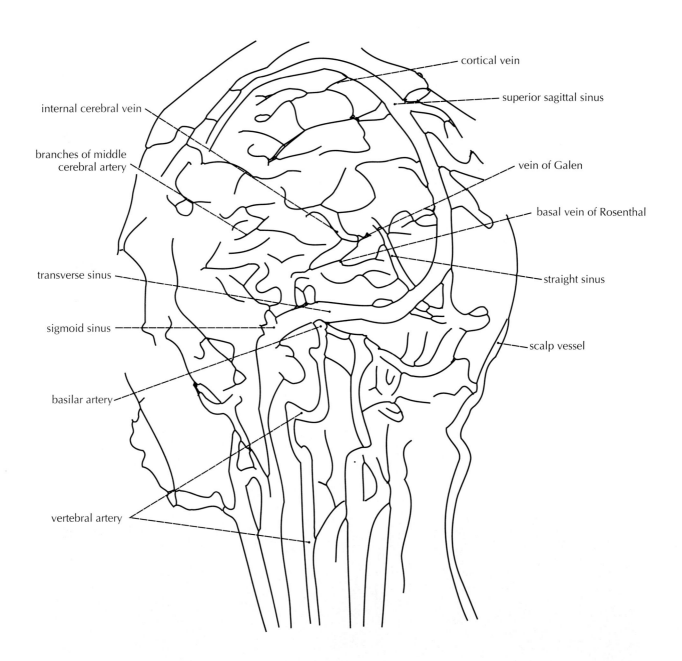

cortical vein

superior sagittal sinus

internal cerebral vein

vein of Galen

branches of middle
cerebral artery

basal vein of Rosenthal

transverse sinus

straight sinus

sigmoid sinus

scalp vessel

basilar artery

vertebral artery

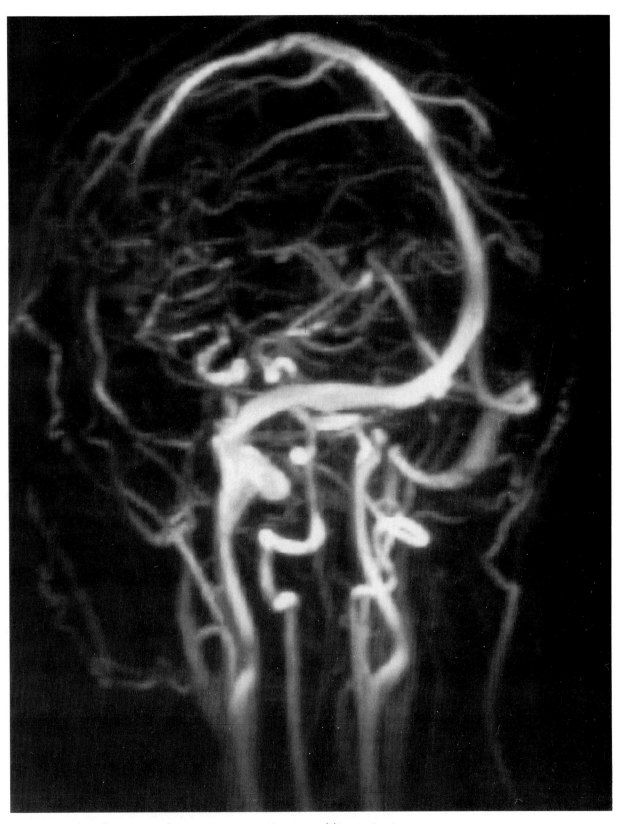

**2-82** Intracranial angiography (noncontrast MR scan, oblique view).

# 2/Sella Turcica, X-Ray

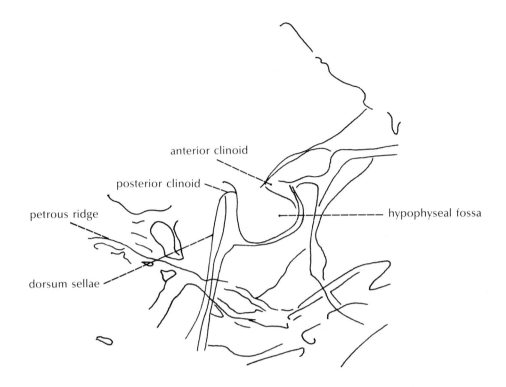

anterior clinoid

posterior clinoid

petrous ridge

dorsum sellae

hypophyseal fossa

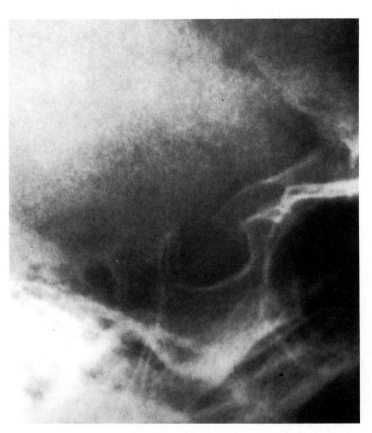

**2-83** Sella turcica, lateral view.

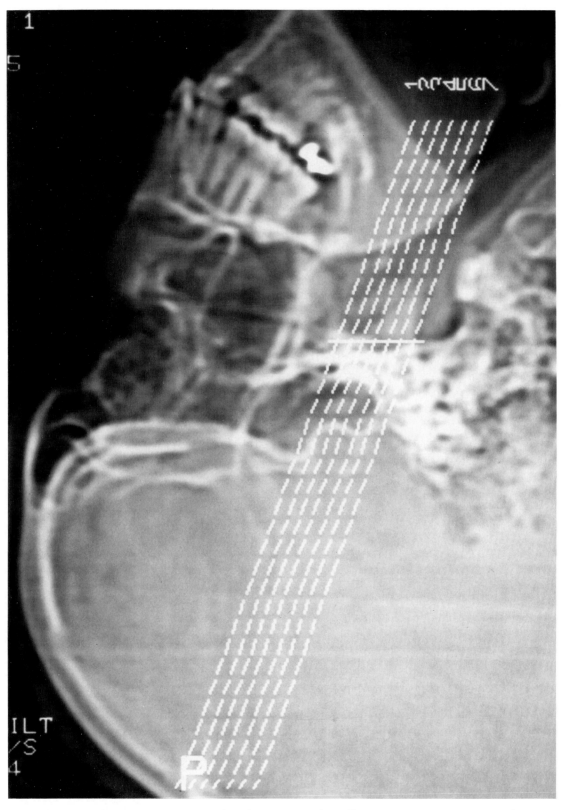

**2-84** This sagittal scout CT scan is used to demonstrate the sellar sections. (Section 3 is used in Figs. 2-85 and 2-86.)

# 2/Sella Turcica, Coronal CT

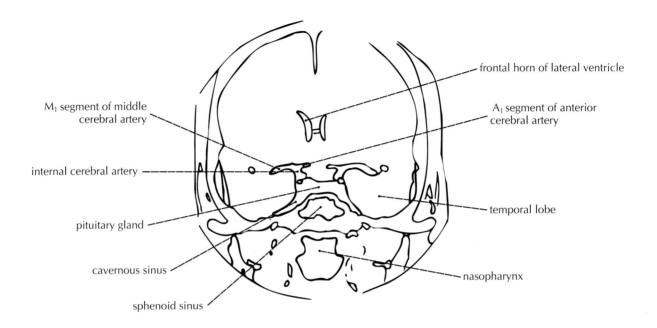

M₁ segment of middle cerebral artery

internal cerebral artery

pituitary gland

cavernous sinus

sphenoid sinus

frontal horn of lateral ventricle

A₁ segment of anterior cerebral artery

temporal lobe

nasopharynx

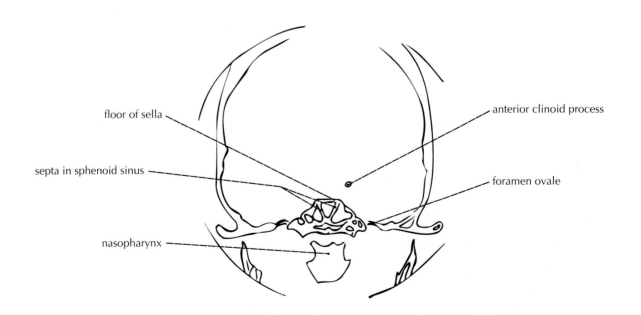

floor of sella

septa in sphenoid sinus

nasopharynx

anterior clinoid process

foramen ovale

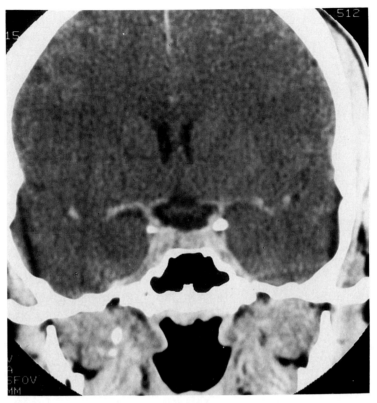

**2-85** Coronal CT scan of pituitary gland with intravenous contrast enhancement.

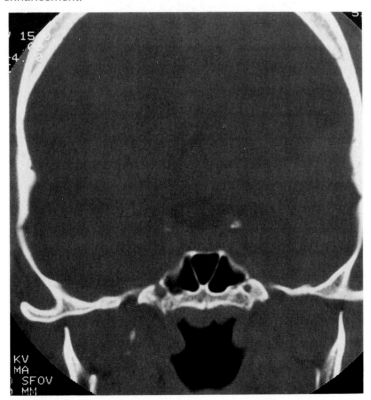

**2-86** Coronal CT scan of pituitary area (same image as Fig. 2-85, but with bone window).

# 2/Sella Turcica, Axial MRI

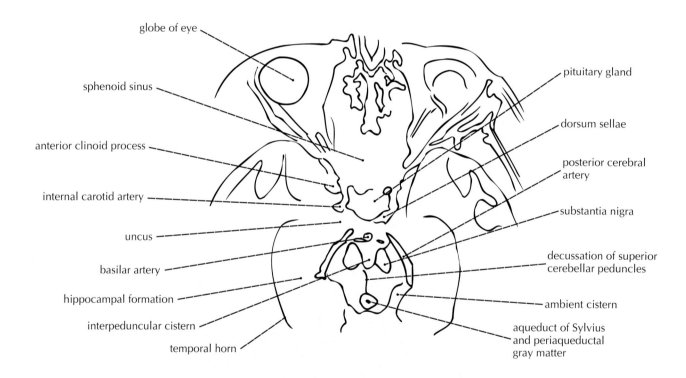

globe of eye

sphenoid sinus

anterior clinoid process

internal carotid artery

uncus

basilar artery

hippocampal formation

interpeduncular cistern

temporal horn

pituitary gland

dorsum sellae

posterior cerebral artery

substantia nigra

decussation of superior cerebellar peduncles

ambient cistern

aqueduct of Sylvius and periaqueductal gray matter

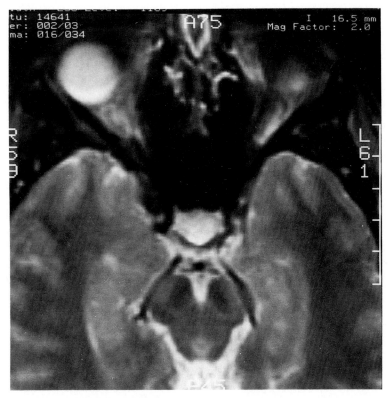

**2-87** Axial MR scan of pituitary gland (2000/90).

# 2/Sella Turcica, Sagittal Scout MRI and Coronal MRI

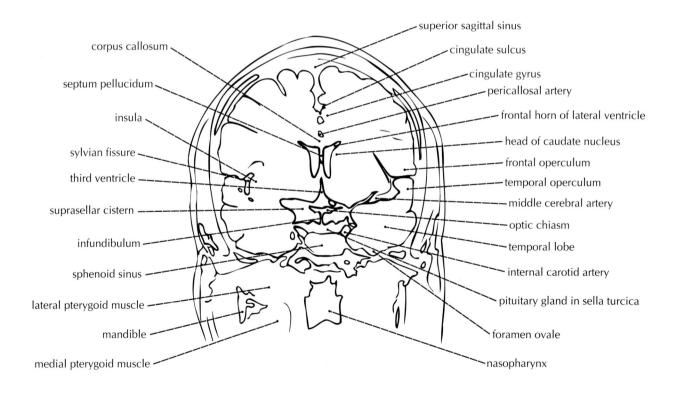

corpus callosum

septum pellucidum

insula

sylvian fissure

third ventricle

suprasellar cistern

infundibulum

sphenoid sinus

lateral pterygoid muscle

mandible

medial pterygoid muscle

superior sagittal sinus

cingulate sulcus

cingulate gyrus

pericallosal artery

frontal horn of lateral ventricle

head of caudate nucleus

frontal operculum

temporal operculum

middle cerebral artery

optic chiasm

temporal lobe

internal carotid artery

pituitary gland in sella turcica

foramen ovale

nasopharynx

# 2/Sella Turcica, Sagittal Scout MRI and Coronal MRI

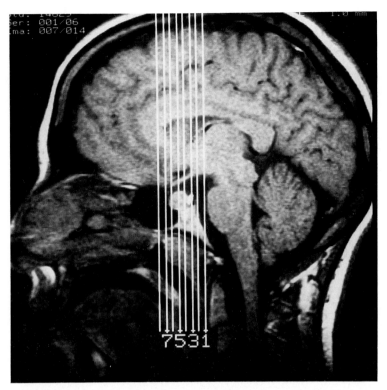

**2-88** This sagittal scout MR scan is used to demonstrate the coronal sections of the pituitary and parapituitary areas. (Sections 6, 5, and 4 are used in Figs. 2-89, 2-90, and 2-91, respectively.)

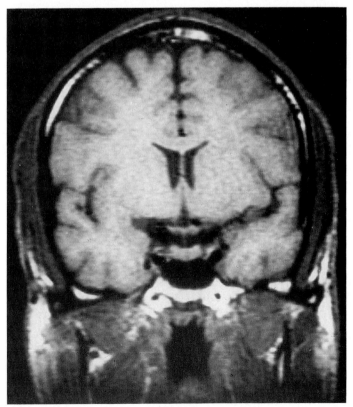

**2-89** Coronal noncontrast MR scan through pituitary gland (section 6 in Fig. 2-88) (600/20).

# 2/Sella Turcica, Coronal MRI

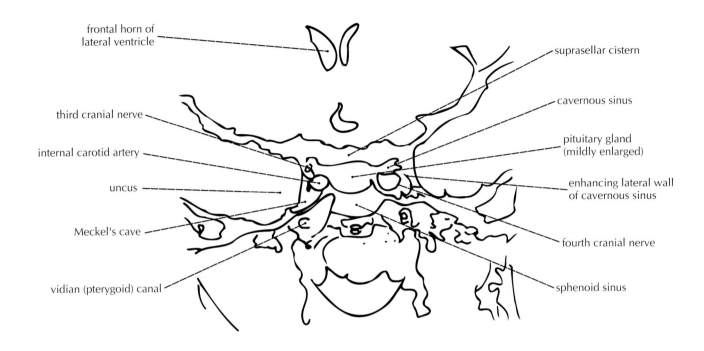

frontal horn of lateral ventricle

third cranial nerve

internal carotid artery

uncus

Meckel's cave

vidian (pterygoid) canal

suprasellar cistern

cavernous sinus

pituitary gland (mildly enlarged)

enhancing lateral wall of cavernous sinus

fourth cranial nerve

sphenoid sinus

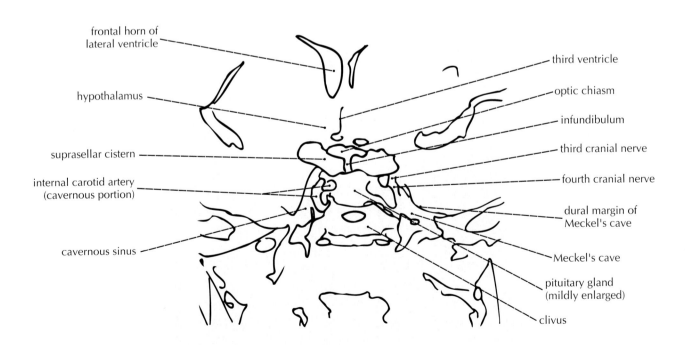

frontal horn of lateral ventricle

hypothalamus

suprasellar cistern

internal carotid artery (cavernous portion)

cavernous sinus

third ventricle

optic chiasm

infundibulum

third cranial nerve

fourth cranial nerve

dural margin of Meckel's cave

Meckel's cave

pituitary gland (mildly enlarged)

clivus

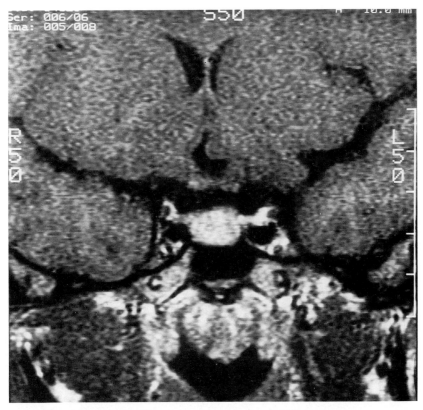

**2-90** Coronal MR scan through pituitary gland with intravenous contrast enhancement (gadolinium-DTPA) (section 5 in Fig. 2-88).

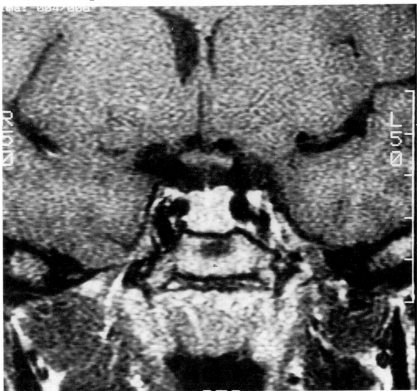

**2-91** Coronal MR scan through pituitary gland with intravenous contrast enhancement (gadolinium-DTPA) (section 4 in Fig. 2-88).

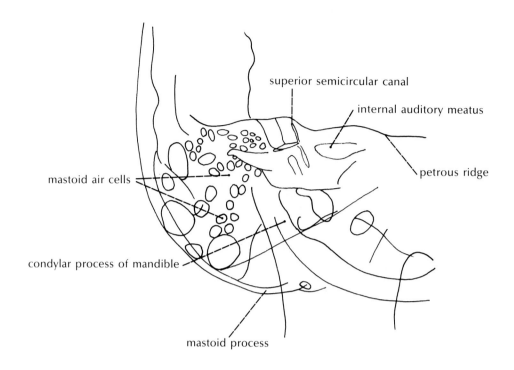

superior semicircular canal

internal auditory meatus

petrous ridge

mastoid air cells

condylar process of mandible

mastoid process

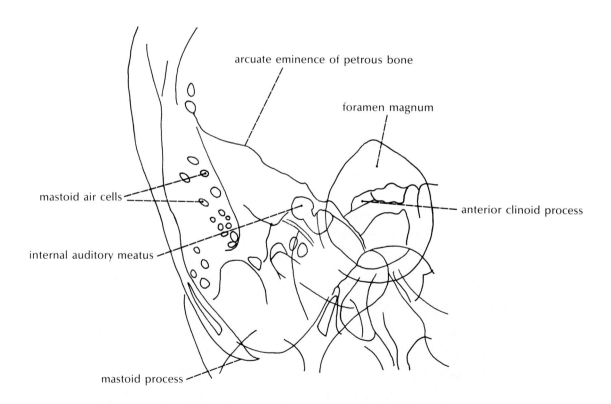

arcuate eminence of petrous bone

foramen magnum

mastoid air cells

anterior clinoid process

internal auditory meatus

mastoid process

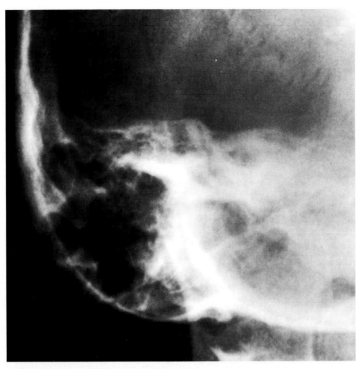

**2-92** Mastoid, Stenvers view.

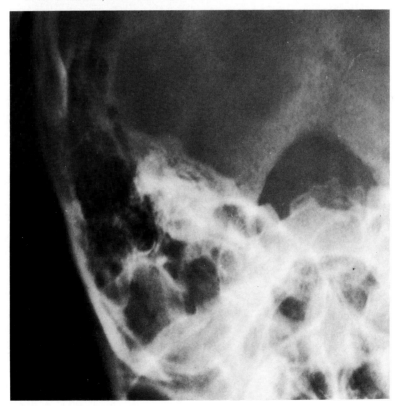

**2-93** Mastoid, Towne view.

# 2/Temporal Bone, Axial CT

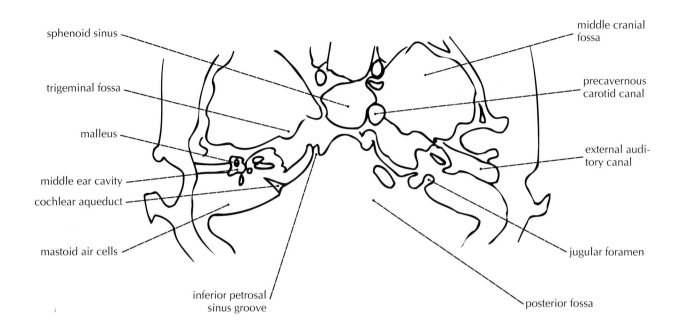

sphenoid sinus

trigeminal fossa

malleus

middle ear cavity

cochlear aqueduct

mastoid air cells

inferior petrosal / sinus groove

middle cranial fossa

precavernous carotid canal

external auditory canal

jugular foramen

posterior fossa

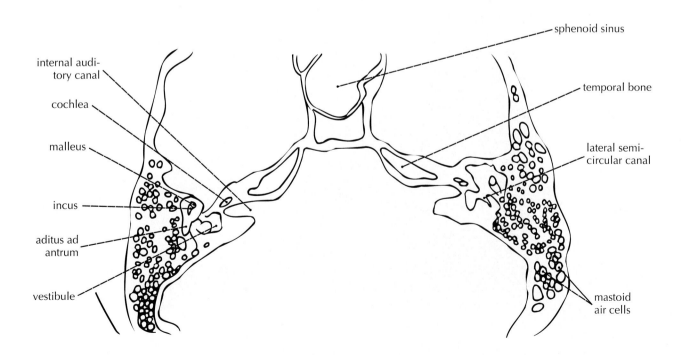

internal auditory canal

cochlea

malleus

incus

aditus ad antrum

vestibule

sphenoid sinus

temporal bone

lateral semicircular canal

mastoid air cells

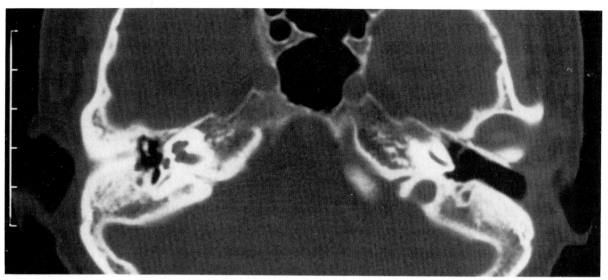

**2-94** Axial CT scan through temporal bone. Section 11 in Fig. 1-6 (p. 13).

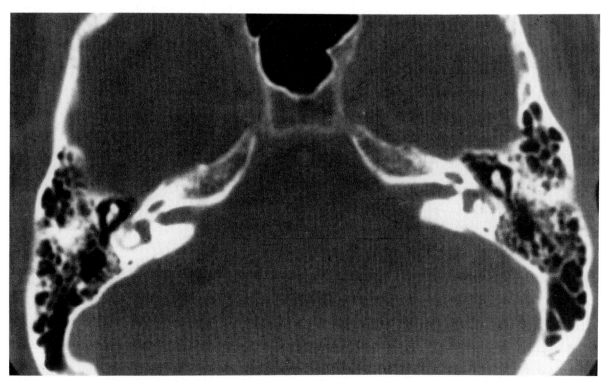

**2-95** Axial CT scan through temporal bone. Section 15 in Fig. 1-6 (p. 13).

# 2/Temporal Bone, Coronal CT

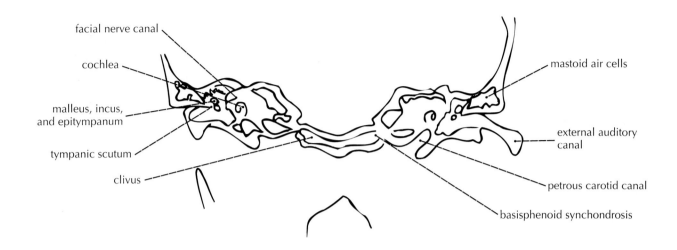

facial nerve canal

cochlea

malleus, incus, and epitympanum

tympanic scutum

clivus

mastoid air cells

external auditory canal

petrous carotid canal

basisphenoid synchondrosis

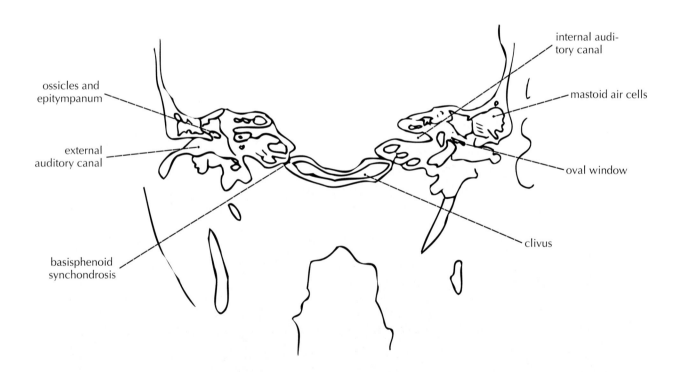

ossicles and epitympanum

external auditory canal

basisphenoid synchondrosis

internal auditory canal

mastoid air cells

oval window

clivus

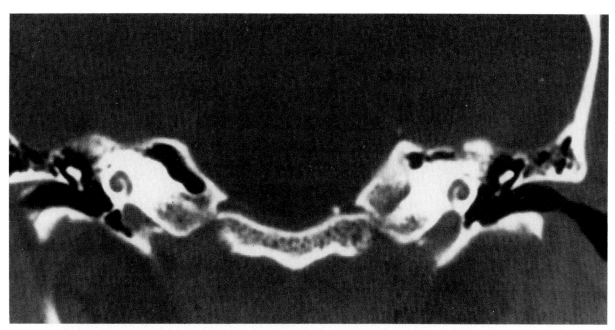

**2-96** Coronal CT scan through skull base. Section 27 in Fig. 1-11 (p. 19).

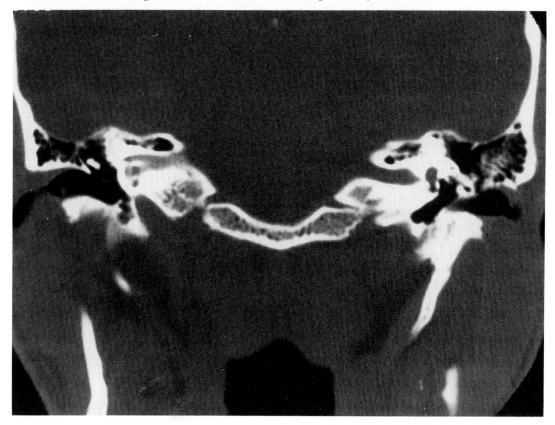

**2-97** Coronal CT scan through skull base and internal auditory canals. Section 7 in Fig. 1-11 (p. 19).

# 2/Temporal Bone, Axial MRI

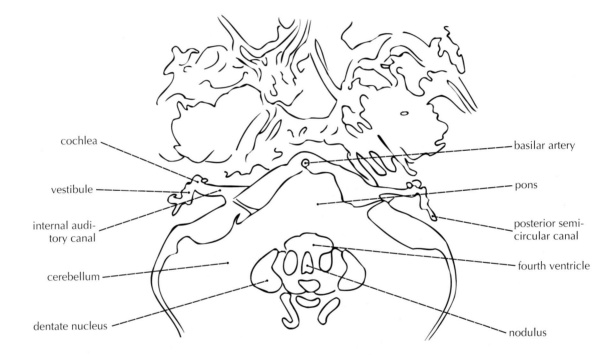

cochlea

vestibule

internal audi-
tory canal

cerebellum

dentate nucleus

basilar artery

pons

posterior semi-
circular canal

fourth ventricle

nodulus

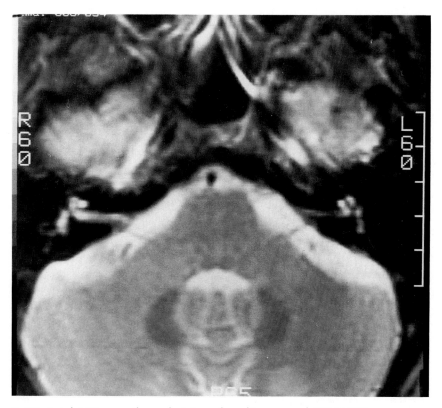

**2-98** Axial MR scan through internal auditory canal (2000/90).

# 2/Temporal Bone, Axial Scout MRI and Coronal MRI

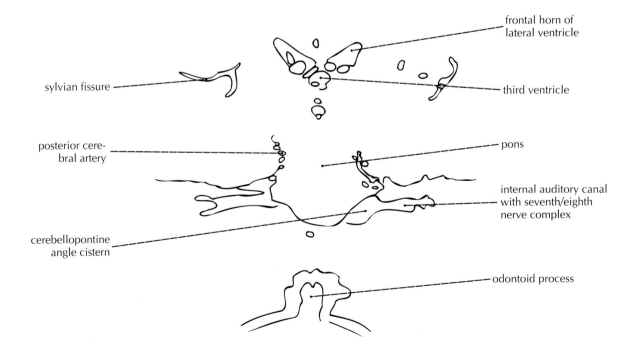

sylvian fissure

frontal horn of
lateral ventricle

third ventricle

posterior cere-
bral artery

pons

internal auditory canal
with seventh/eighth
nerve complex

cerebellopontine
angle cistern

odontoid process

# 2/Temporal Bone, Axial Scout MRI and Coronal MRI

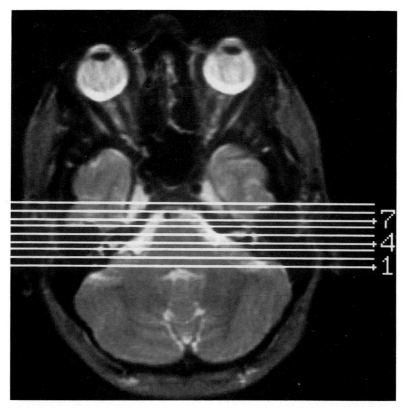

**2-99** Axial scout MRI for the coronal MRI.

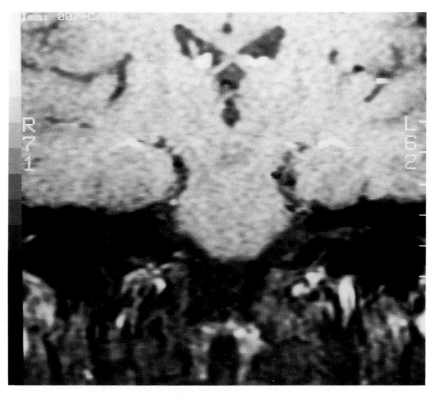

**2-100** Coronal MR scan through internal auditory canal (gadolinium-DTPA–enhanced study) (600/20). Section 5 in Fig. 2-99.

# PART 2

# THE NECK AND SPINE

# 3/**Cervical Spine** □ Cervical Spine, X-Ray

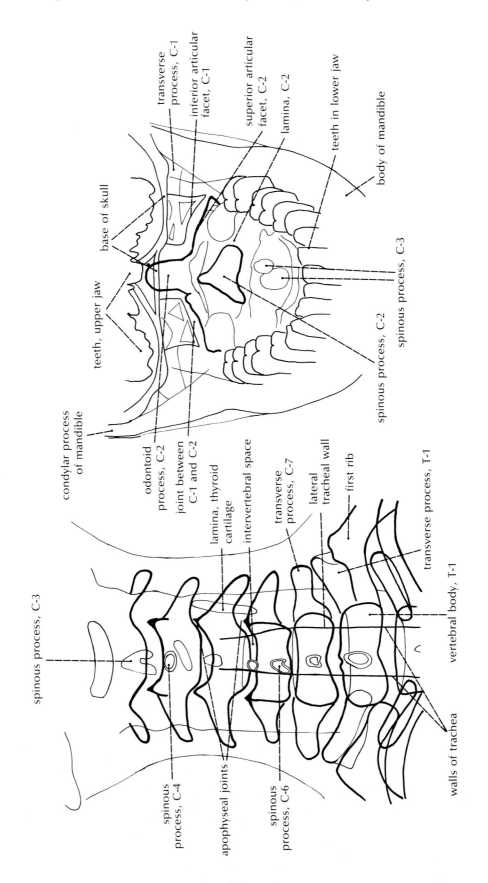

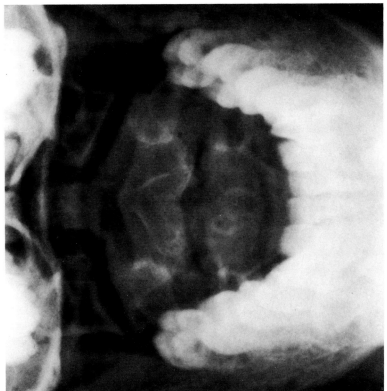

3-2 Cervical spine, open-mouth view.

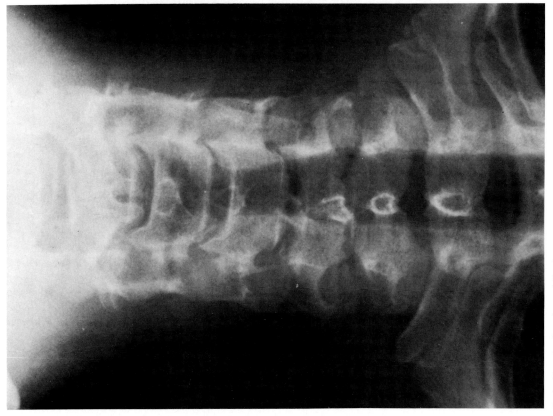

3-1 Cervical spine, AP view.

# 3/Cervical Spine, X-Ray

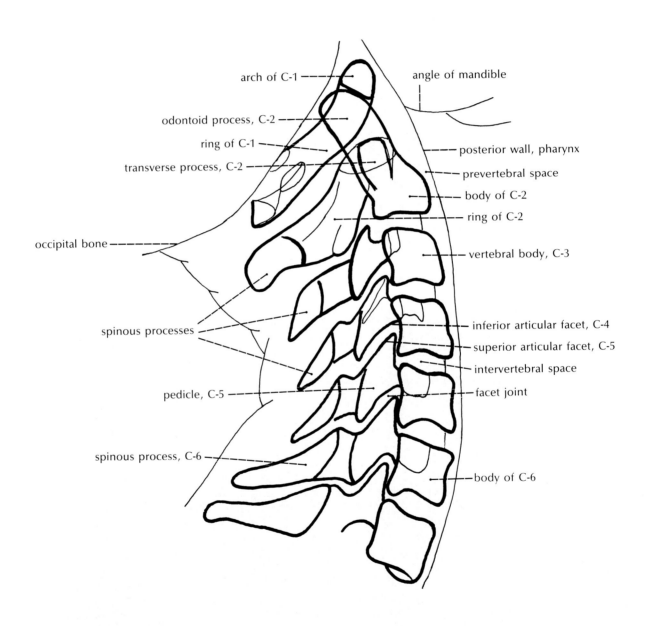

arch of C-1

odontoid process, C-2

ring of C-1

transverse process, C-2

occipital bone

spinous processes

pedicle, C-5

spinous process, C-6

angle of mandible

posterior wall, pharynx

prevertebral space

body of C-2

ring of C-2

vertebral body, C-3

inferior articular facet, C-4

superior articular facet, C-5

intervertebral space

facet joint

body of C-6

# 3/Cervical Spine, X-Ray

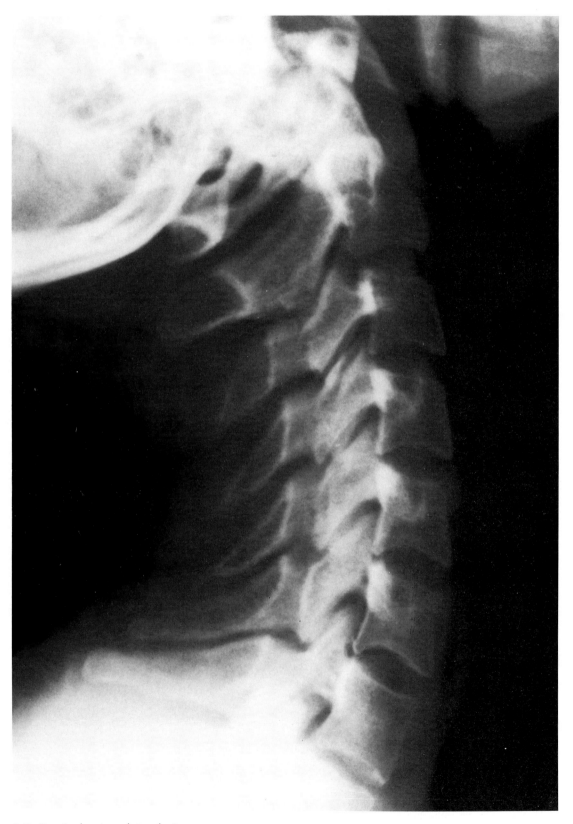

**3-3** Cervical spine, lateral view.

# 3/Cervical Spine, X-Ray

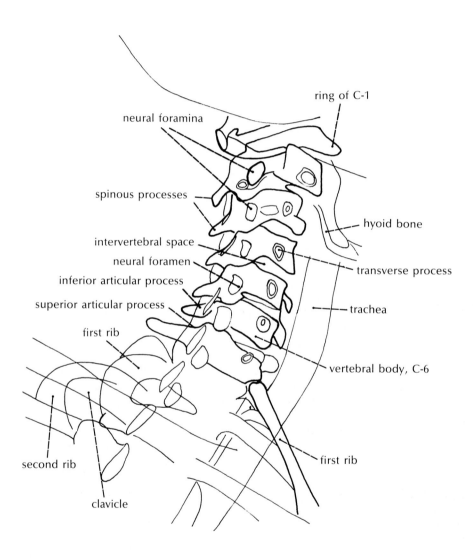

neural foramina

ring of C-1

spinous processes

hyoid bone

intervertebral space

neural foramen

transverse process

inferior articular process

superior articular process

trachea

first rib

vertebral body, C-6

second rib

first rib

clavicle

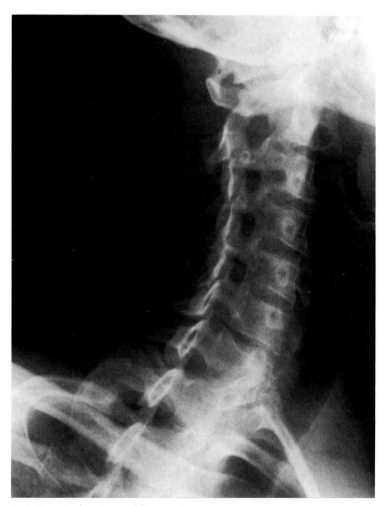

**3-4** Cervical spine, oblique view.

# 3/Cervical Spine, Sagittal Scout CT and Axial CT

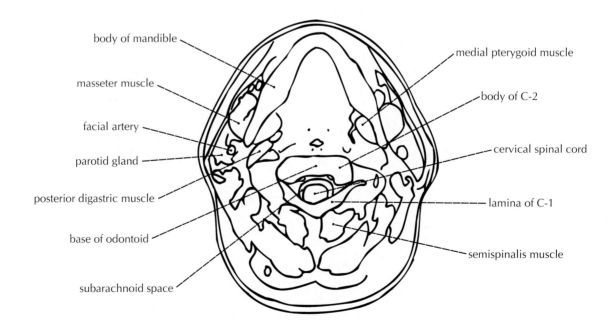

body of mandible

masseter muscle

facial artery

parotid gland

posterior digastric muscle

base of odontoid

subarachnoid space

medial pterygoid muscle

body of C-2

cervical spinal cord

lamina of C-1

semispinalis muscle

# 3/Cervical Spine, Sagittal Scout CT and Axial CT

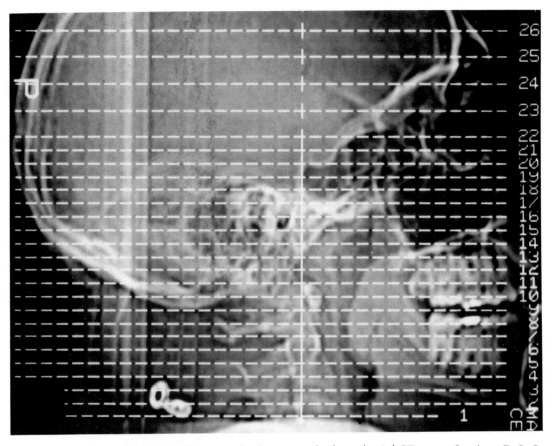

**3-5** This sagittal scout CT scan illustrates the location of selected axial CT scans. Sections 7, 2, 9, and 3 are shown.

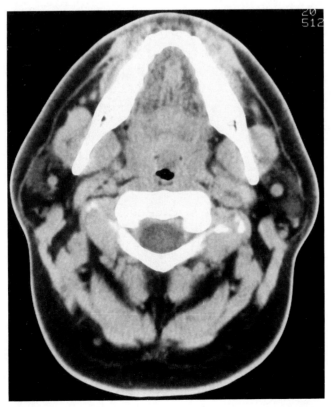

**3-6** Axial CT scan through body of C-2. Section 7 in Fig. 3-5.

# 3/Cervical Spine, Axial CT

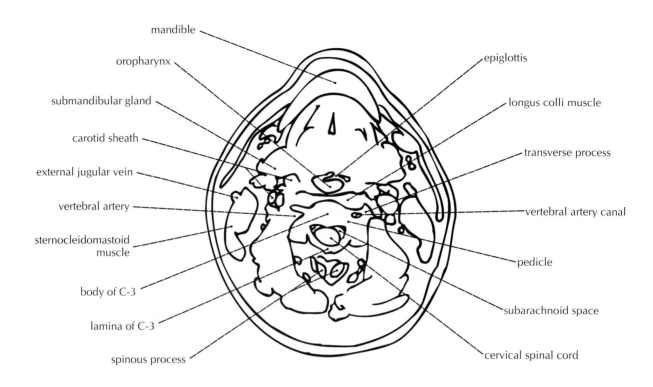

mandible

oropharynx

submandibular gland

carotid sheath

external jugular vein

vertebral artery

sternocleidomastoid
muscle

body of C-3

lamina of C-3

spinous process

epiglottis

longus colli muscle

transverse process

vertebral artery canal

pedicle

subarachnoid space

cervical spinal cord

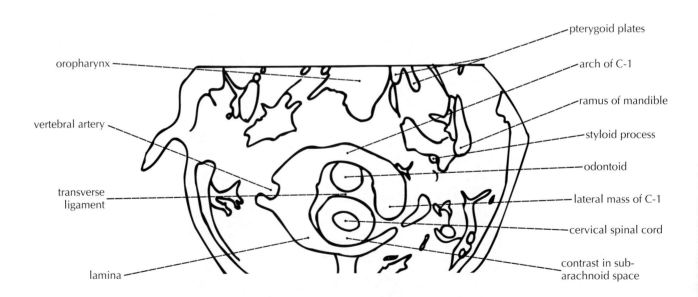

oropharynx

vertebral artery

transverse
ligament

lamina

pterygoid plates

arch of C-1

ramus of mandible

styloid process

odontoid

lateral mass of C-1

cervical spinal cord

contrast in sub-
arachnoid space

# 3/Cervical Spine, Axial CT

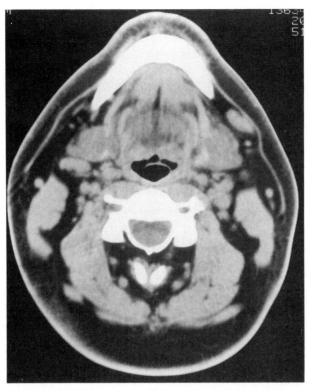

**3-7** Axial CT scan through body of C-3. Section 2 in Fig. 3-5.

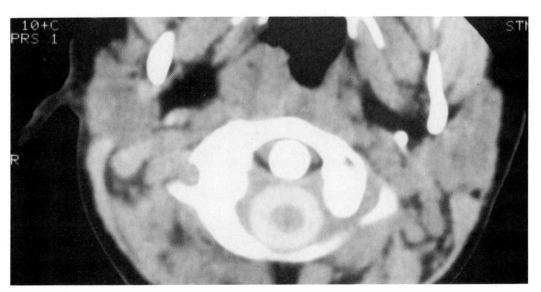

**3-8** Axial CT scan through cervical spine (with intrathecal contrast) at C-1–C-2 level. Section 9 in Fig. 3-5.

# 3/Cervical Spine, Axial CT

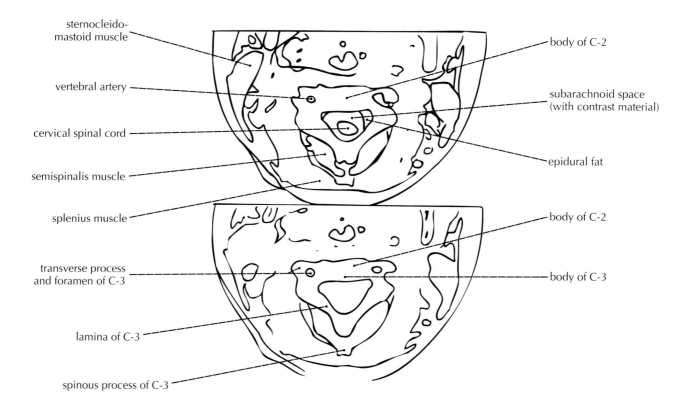

sternocleido-
mastoid muscle

vertebral artery

cervical spinal cord

semispinalis muscle

splenius muscle

transverse process
and foramen of C-3

lamina of C-3

spinous process of C-3

body of C-2

subarachnoid space
(with contrast material)

epidural fat

body of C-2

body of C-3

# 3/Cervical Spine, Axial CT

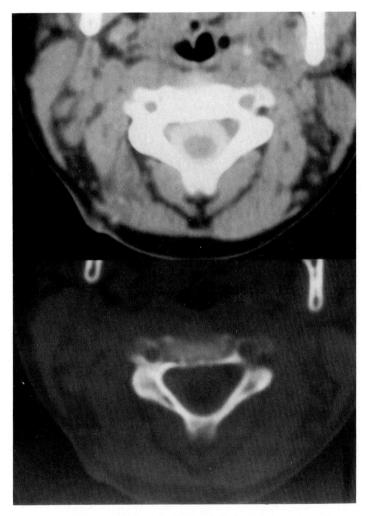

**3-9** Axial CT scans through C-2 and C-3 with intrathecal contrast (soft tissue and bone window). Section 3 in Fig. 3-5.

# 3/Cervical Spine, Sagittal and Parasagittal MRI

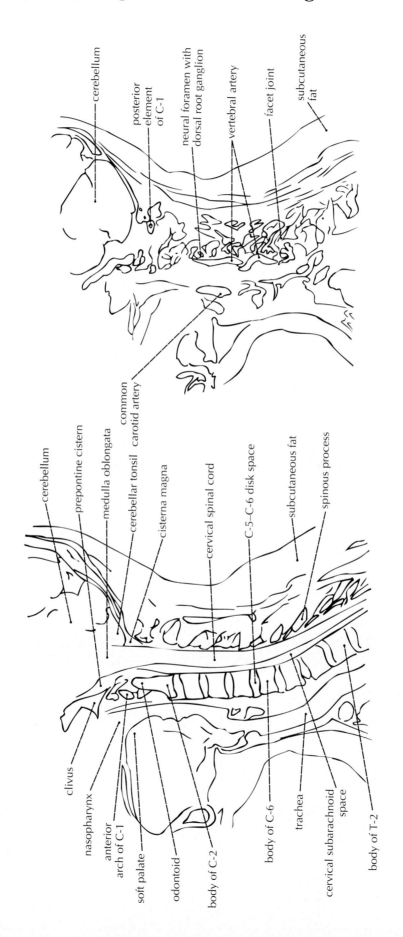

# 3/Cervical Spine, Sagittal and Parasagittal MRI

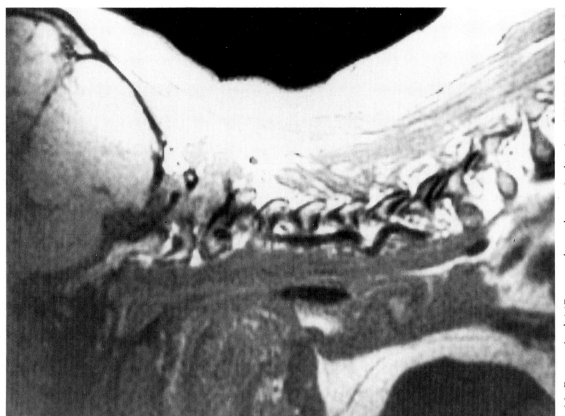

**3-11** Parasagittal MR scan through cervical spine (600/20). Section is 1.5 cm lateral to midline.

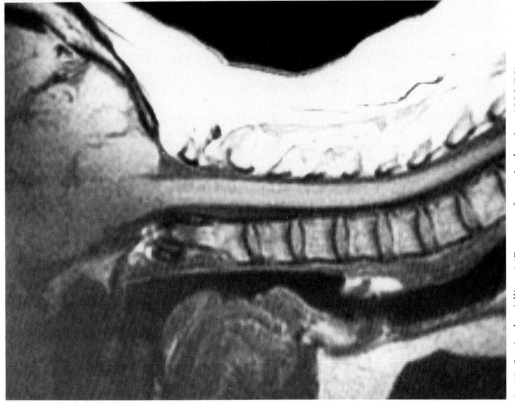

**3-10** Sagittal midline MR scan of cervical spine (600/20).

# 3/Cervical Spine, Sagittal MRI

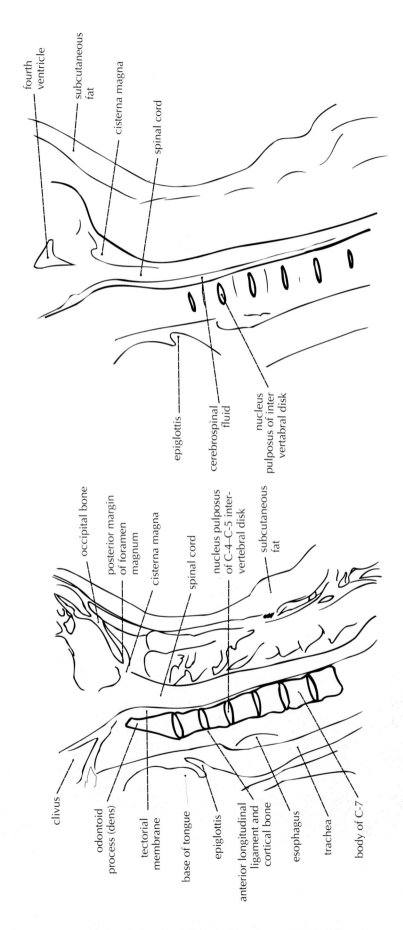

fourth ventricle

subcutaneous fat

cisterna magna

spinal cord

epiglottis

cerebrospinal fluid

nucleus pulposus of inter vertabral disk

occipital bone

posterior margin of foramen magnum

cisterna magna

spinal cord

nucleus pulposus of C-4–C-5 inter- vertebral disk

subcutaneous fat

clivus

odontoid process (dens)

tectorial membrane

base of tongue

epiglottis

anterior longitudinal ligament and cortical bone

esophagus

trachea

body of C-7

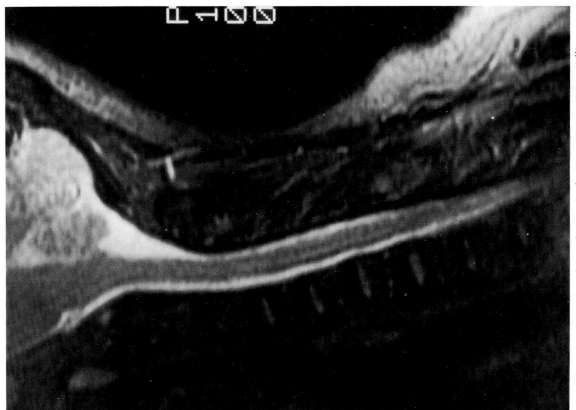

**3-13** Sagittal MR scan through cervical spine (2000/90). Midline section.

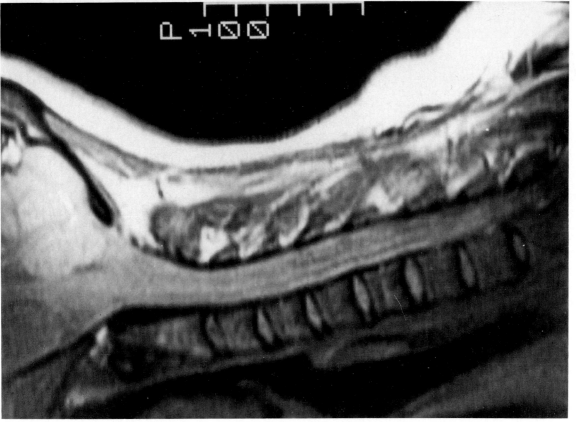

**3-12** Sagittal MR scan through cervical spine (2000/30). Midline section.

# 3/Cervical Spine, Sagittal Scout MRI and Axial MRI

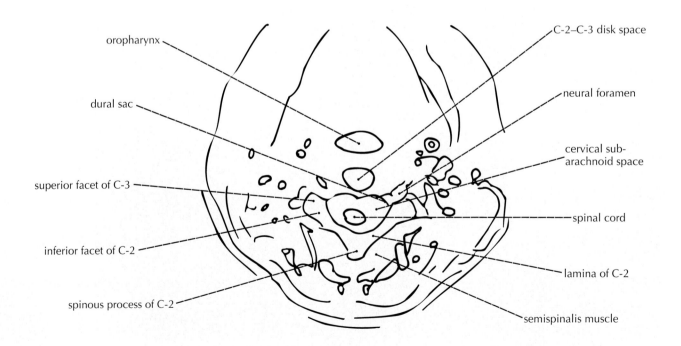

oropharynx

C-2–C-3 disk space

neural foramen

dural sac

cervical sub-
arachnoid space

superior facet of C-3

spinal cord

inferior facet of C-2

lamina of C-2

spinous process of C-2

semispinalis muscle

# 3/Cervical Spine, Sagittal Scout MRI and Axial MRI

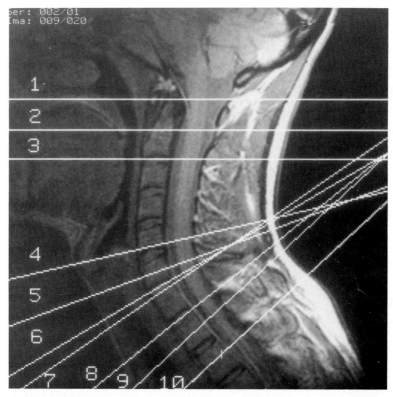

**3-14** Sagittal scout MR scan of cervical spine for orientation of selected axial MR scans. Sections 3, 4, and 7 will be shown.

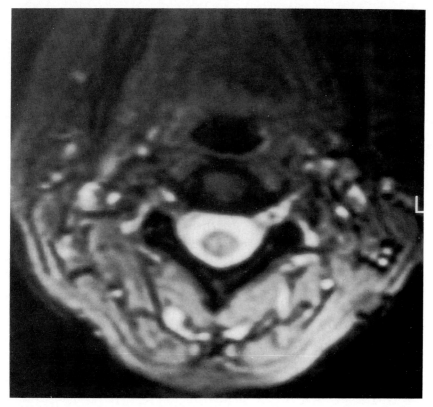

**3-15** Axial MR scan through C-2–C-3 level (500/18, flip angle 15°) (section 3 in Fig. 3-14).

# 3/Cervical Spine, Axial MRI

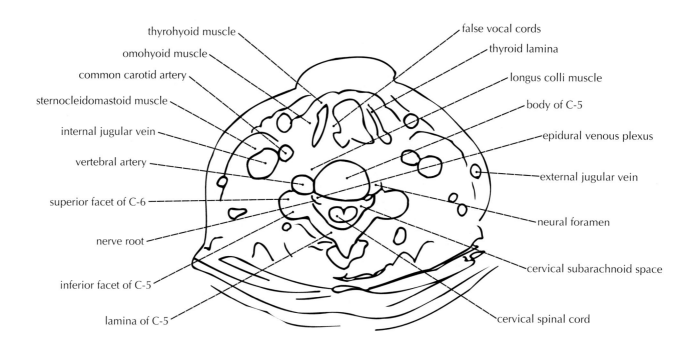

thyrohyoid muscle
omohyoid muscle
common carotid artery
sternocleidomastoid muscle
internal jugular vein
vertebral artery
superior facet of C-6
nerve root
inferior facet of C-5
lamina of C-5

false vocal cords
thyroid lamina
longus colli muscle
body of C-5
epidural venous plexus
external jugular vein
neural foramen
cervical subarachnoid space
cervical spinal cord

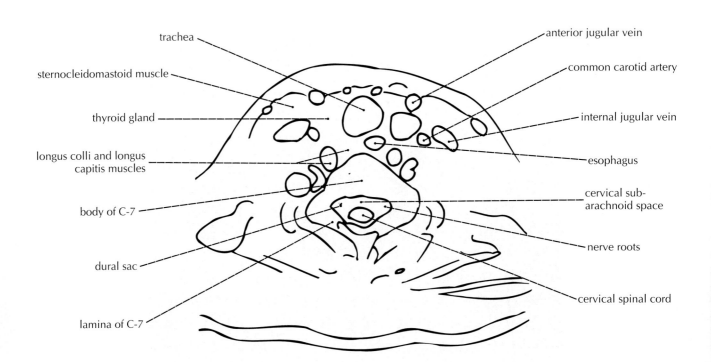

trachea
sternocleidomastoid muscle
thyroid gland
longus colli and longus capitis muscles
body of C-7
dural sac
lamina of C-7

anterior jugular vein
common carotid artery
internal jugular vein
esophagus
cervical sub-arachnoid space
nerve roots
cervical spinal cord

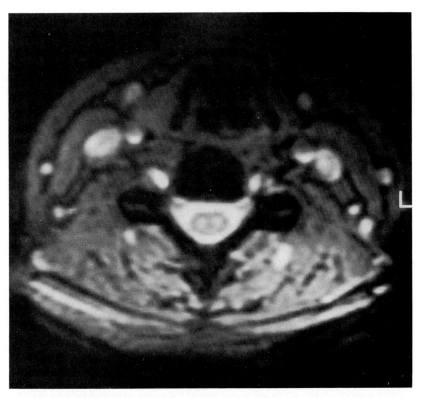

**3-16** Axial MR scan through body of C-5 (500/18, flip angle 15°) (section 4 in Fig. 3-14).

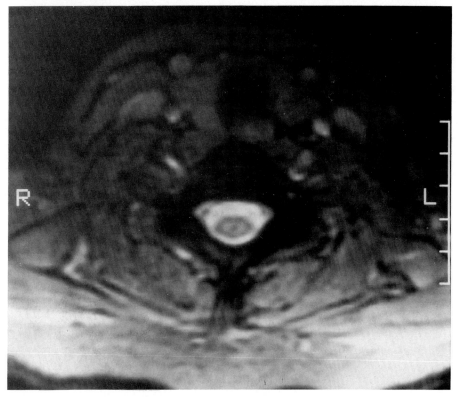

**3-17** Axial MR scan through body of C-7 (500/18, flip angle 15°) (section 7 in Fig. 3-14).

# 3/Cervical Spine, Axial MRI

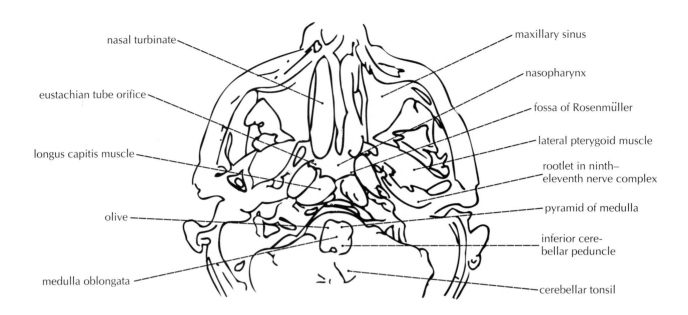

nasal turbinate

eustachian tube orifice

longus capitis muscle

olive

medulla oblongata

maxillary sinus

nasopharynx

fossa of Rosenmüller

lateral pterygoid muscle

rootlet in ninth–eleventh nerve complex

pyramid of medulla

inferior cere-bellar peduncle

cerebellar tonsil

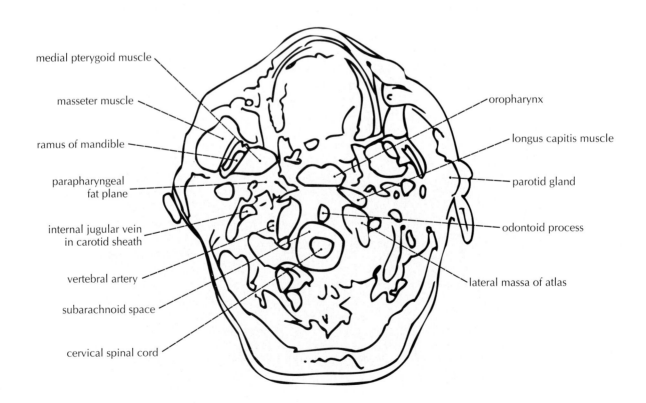

medial pterygoid muscle

masseter muscle

ramus of mandible

parapharyngeal fat plane

internal jugular vein in carotid sheath

vertebral artery

subarachnoid space

cervical spinal cord

oropharynx

longus capitis muscle

parotid gland

odontoid process

lateral massa of atlas

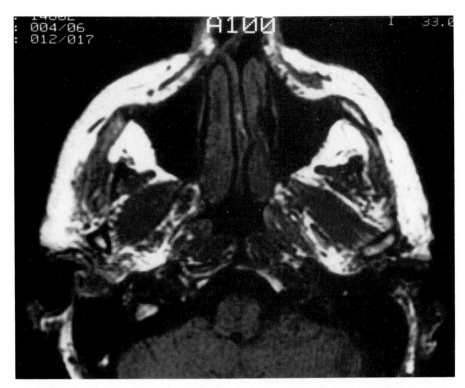

**3-18** Axial MR scan through medulla and nasopharynx (600/20). Section 6 in Fig. 2-12.

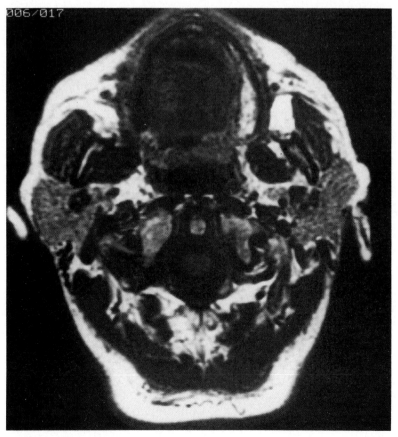

**3-19** Axial MR scan through C-1–C-2 (600/15). Section 1 in Fig. 3-14.

# 3/Cervical Spine, Axial MRI

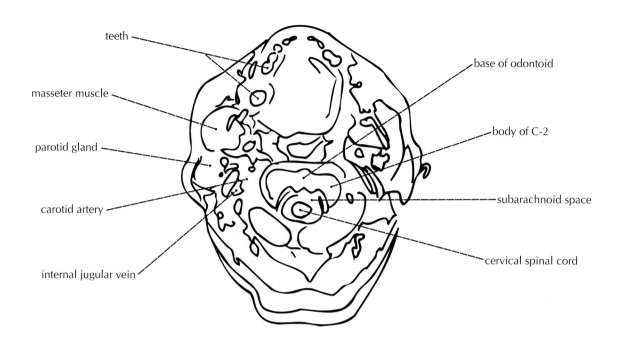

teeth

masseter muscle

parotid gland

carotid artery

internal jugular vein

base of odontoid

body of C-2

subarachnoid space

cervical spinal cord

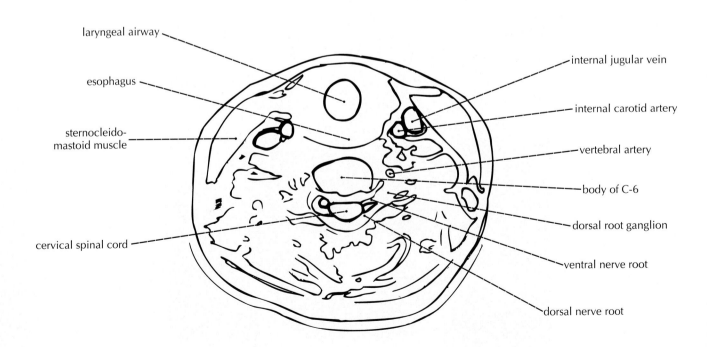

laryngeal airway

esophagus

sternocleido-mastoid muscle

cervical spinal cord

internal jugular vein

internal carotid artery

vertebral artery

body of C-6

dorsal root ganglion

ventral nerve root

dorsal nerve root

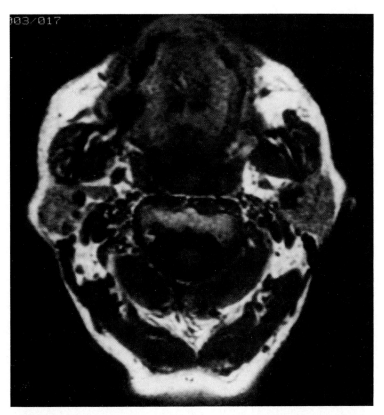

**3-20** Axial MR scan through body of C-2 (600/15). Section 2 in Fig. 3-14.

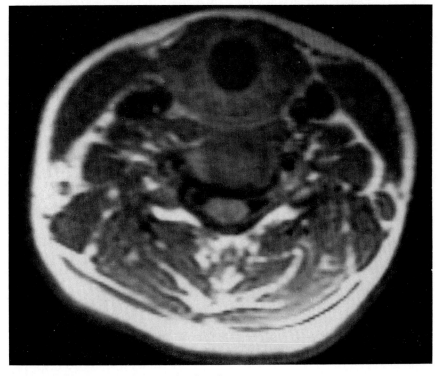

**3-21** Axial MR scan through body of C-6 (800/20) (section 5 in Fig. 3-14).

# 3/Cervical Spine, Axial MRI

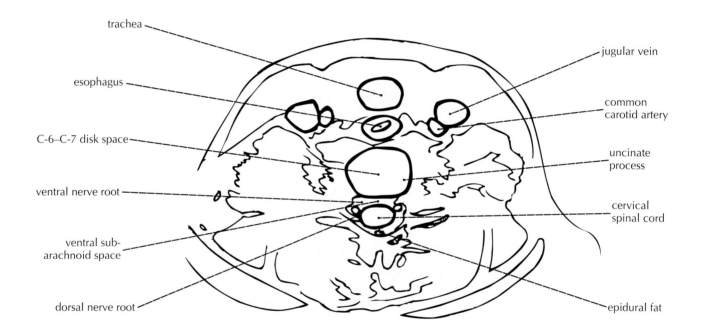

trachea

jugular vein

esophagus

common
carotid artery

C-6–C-7 disk space

uncinate
process

ventral nerve root

cervical
spinal cord

ventral sub-
arachnoid space

dorsal nerve root

epidural fat

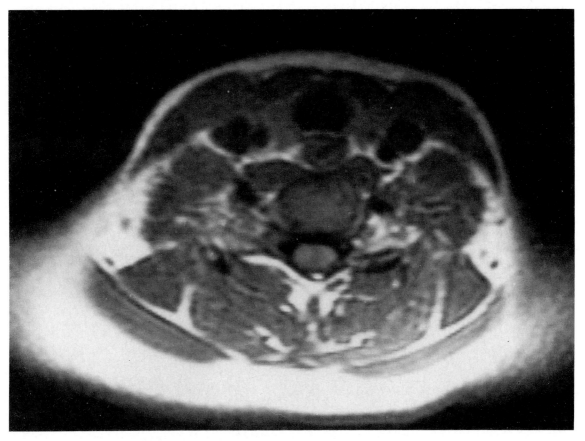

**3-22** Axial MR scan through C-6–C-7 disk space (800/20) (section 6 in Fig. 3-14).

# 3/Neck, Arteriography

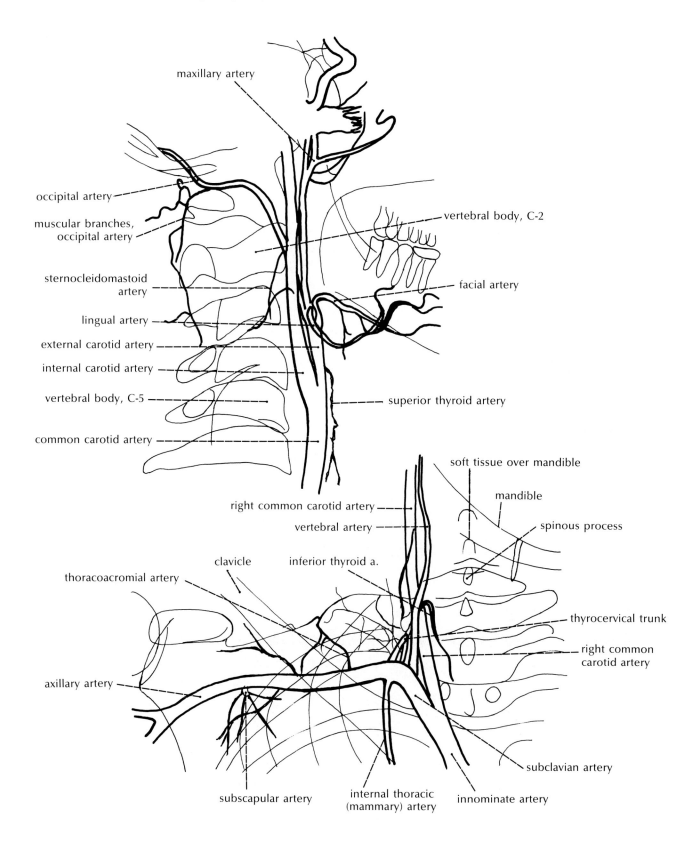

maxillary artery

occipital artery

muscular branches, occipital artery

vertebral body, C-2

sternocleidomastoid artery

facial artery

lingual artery

external carotid artery

internal carotid artery

vertebral body, C-5

superior thyroid artery

common carotid artery

soft tissue over mandible

mandible

right common carotid artery

vertebral artery

spinous process

clavicle

inferior thyroid a.

thoracoacromial artery

thyrocervical trunk

right common carotid artery

axillary artery

subscapular artery

internal thoracic (mammary) artery

innominate artery

subclavian artery

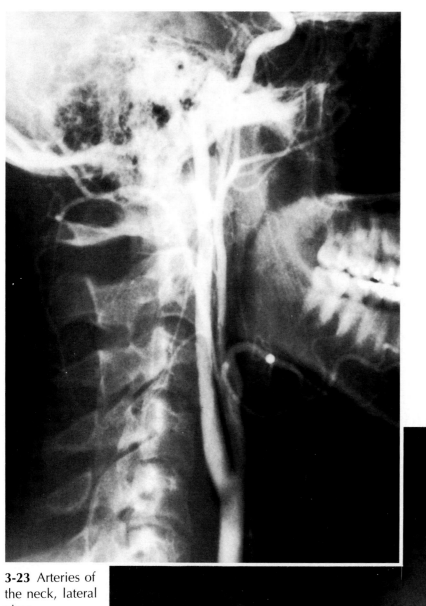

**3-23** Arteries of the neck, lateral view.

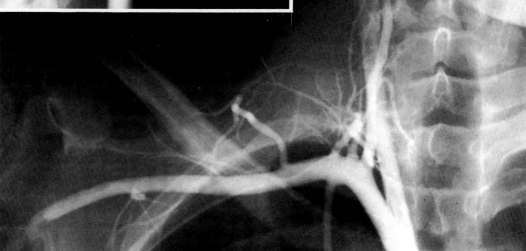

**3-24** Arteries of the neck, AP view.

# 3/Neck, Angiography

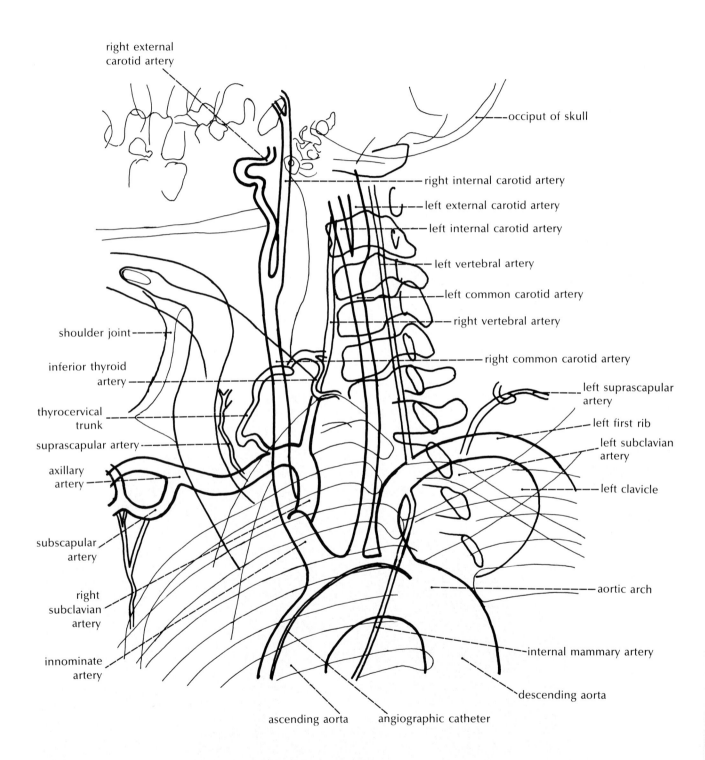

right external carotid artery

occiput of skull

right internal carotid artery

left external carotid artery

left internal carotid artery

left vertebral artery

left common carotid artery

right vertebral artery

shoulder joint

right common carotid artery

inferior thyroid artery

left suprascapular artery

left first rib

thyrocervical trunk

left subclavian artery

suprascapular artery

left clavicle

axillary artery

subscapular artery

aortic arch

right subclavian artery

internal mammary artery

innominate artery

descending aorta

ascending aorta

angiographic catheter

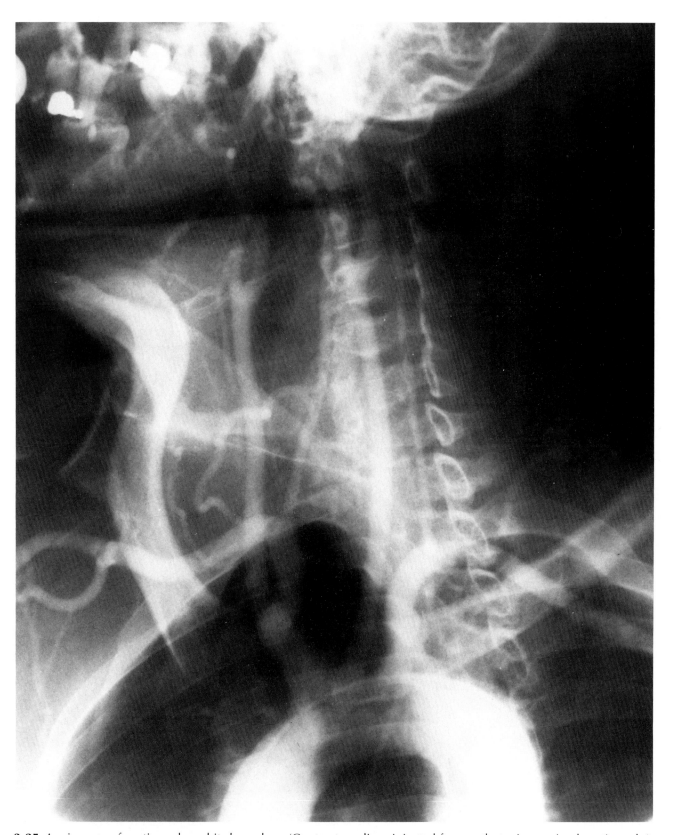

**3-25** Angiogram of aortic arch and its branches. (Contrast medium injected from catheter in proximal aortic arch.)

# 3/Neck, MR Angiography

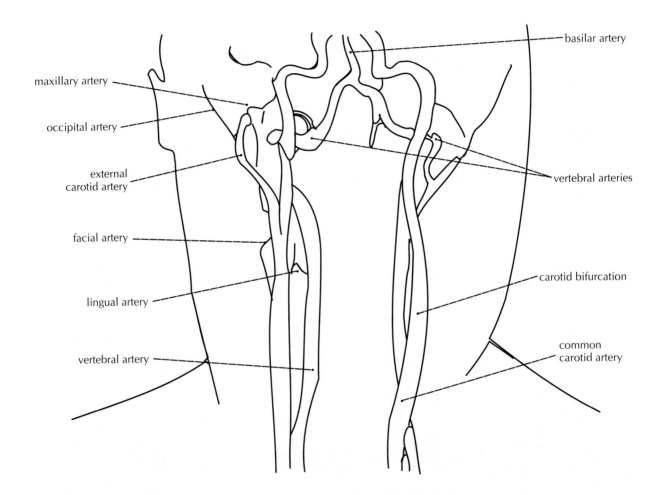

maxillary artery

occipital artery

external
carotid artery

facial artery

lingual artery

vertebral artery

basilar artery

vertebral arteries

carotid bifurcation

common
carotid artery

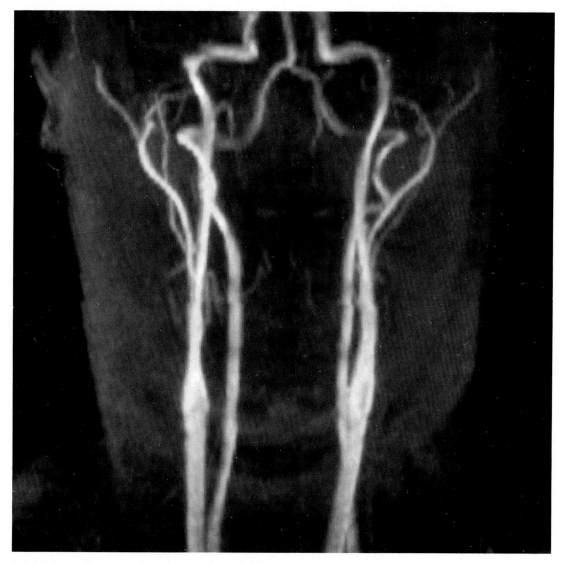

**3-26** MR angiogram of neck vessels, frontal view (noncontrast study).

# 3/Neck, MR Angiography

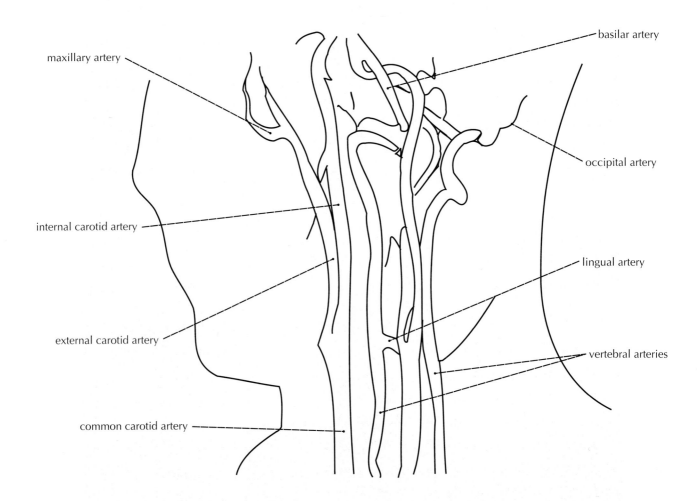

maxillary artery

basilar artery

occipital artery

internal carotid artery

lingual artery

external carotid artery

vertebral arteries

common carotid artery

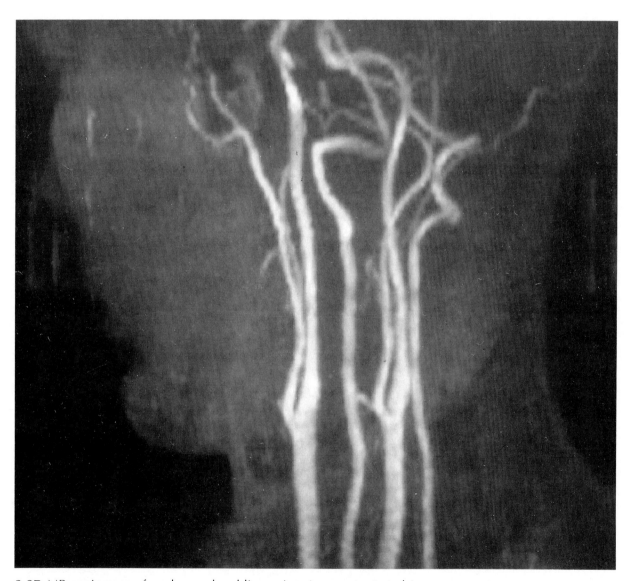

**3-27** MR angiogram of neck vessels, oblique view (noncontrast study).

# 3/Cervical Spine, Myelography

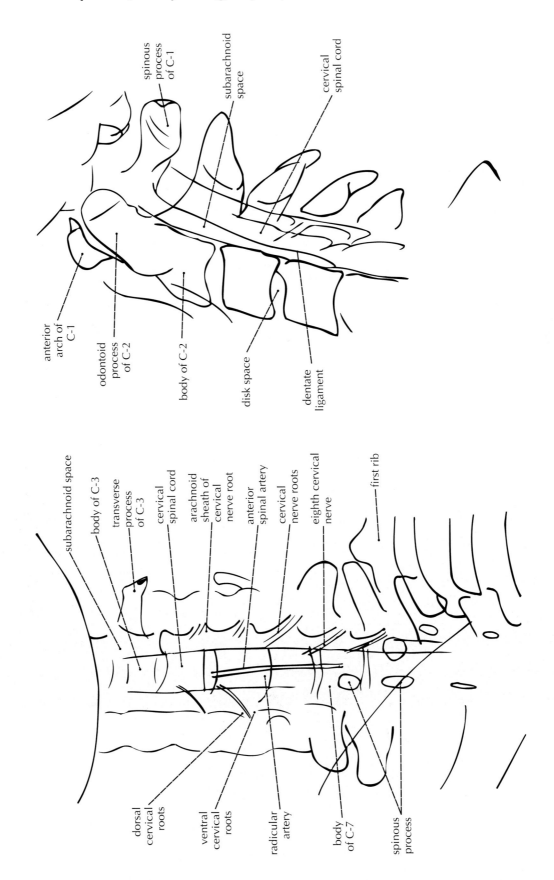

spinous process of C-1

subarachnoid space

cervical spinal cord

anterior arch of C-1

odontoid process of C-2

body of C-2

disk space

dentate ligament

subarachnoid space

body of C-3

transverse process of C-3

cervical spinal cord

arachnoid sheath of cervical nerve root

anterior spinal artery

cervical nerve roots

eighth cervical nerve

first rib

dorsal cervical roots

ventral cervical roots

radicular artery

body of C-7

spinous process

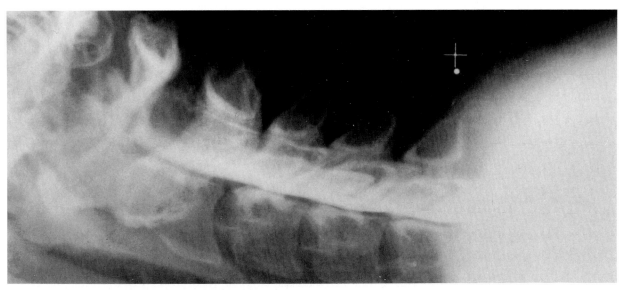

3-29 Cervical myelogram, lateral view.

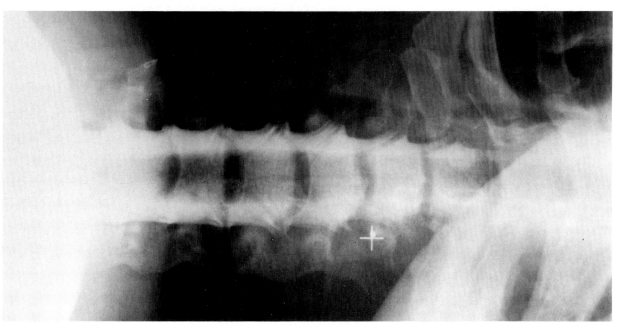

3-28 Cervical myelogram, AP view.

# 3/Cervical Spine, Myelography

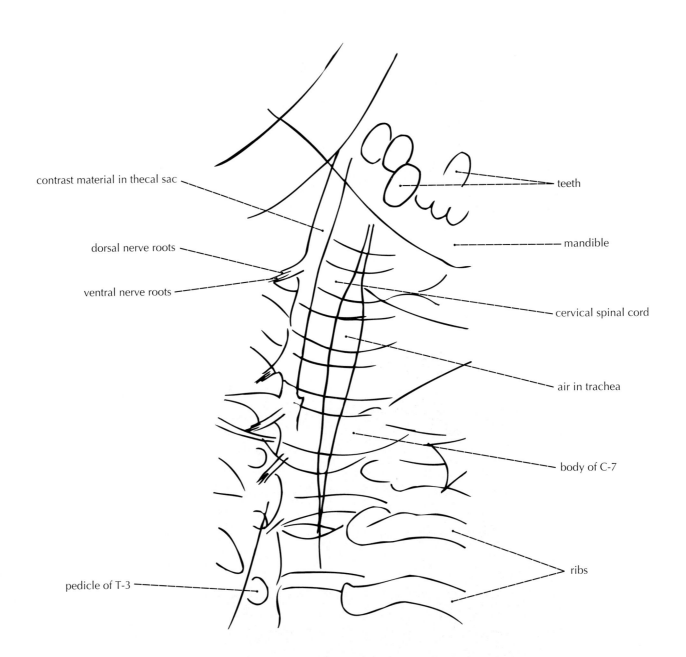

contrast material in thecal sac

dorsal nerve roots

ventral nerve roots

pedicle of T-3

teeth

mandible

cervical spinal cord

air in trachea

body of C-7

ribs

# 3/Cervical Spine, Myelography

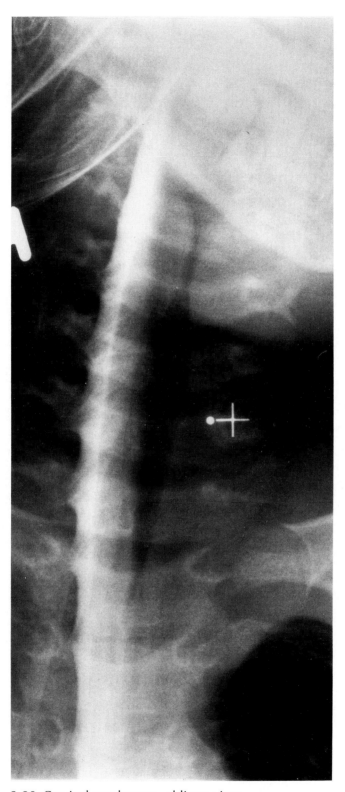

**3-30** Cervical myelogram, oblique view.

# 4/**Thoracic Spine** □ Thoracic Spine, X-Ray

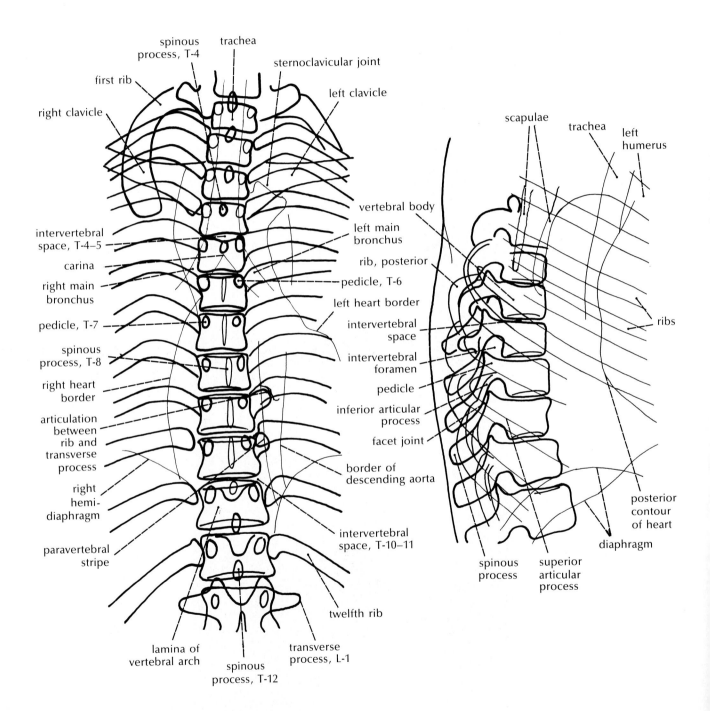

spinous process, T-4

trachea

first rib

sternoclavicular joint

right clavicle

left clavicle

vertebral body

left main bronchus

intervertebral space, T-4–5

carina

rib, posterior

pedicle, T-6

right main bronchus

left heart border

pedicle, T-7

intervertebral space

spinous process, T-8

intervertebral foramen

right heart border

pedicle

articulation between rib and transverse process

inferior articular process

facet joint

right hemi-diaphragm

border of descending aorta

paravertebral stripe

intervertebral space, T-10–11

twelfth rib

lamina of vertebral arch

spinous process, T-12

transverse process, L-1

scapulae

trachea

left humerus

ribs

posterior contour of heart

diaphragm

spinous process

superior articular process

# 4/Thoracic Spine, X-Ray

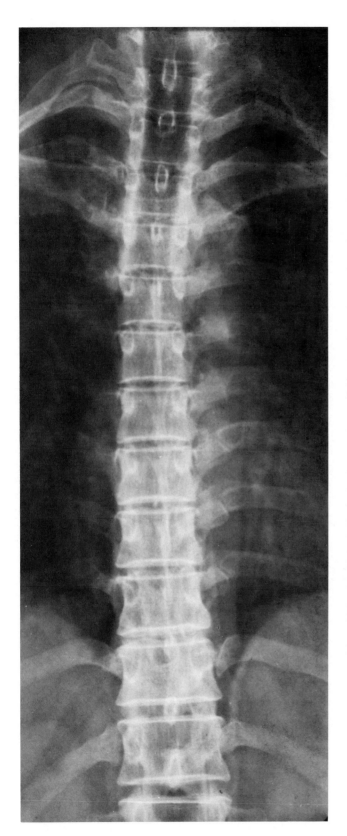

**4-1** Thoracic spine, AP view.

**4-2** Thoracic spine, lateral view.

# 4/Thoracic Spine, Sagittal Scout CT and Axial CT

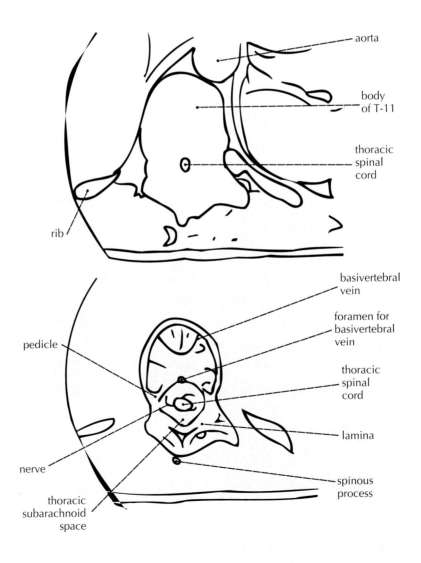

aorta

body of T-11

thoracic spinal cord

rib

basivertebral vein

foramen for basivertebral vein

thoracic spinal cord

lamina

spinous process

pedicle

nerve

thoracic subarachnoid space

# 4/Thoracic Spine, Sagittal Scout CT and Axial CT

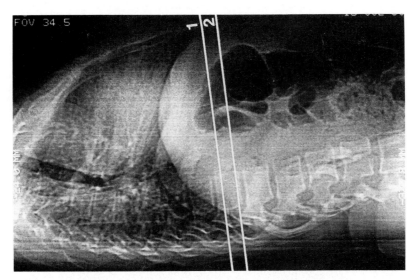

**4-3** Sagittal scout CT for demonstration of the axial images.

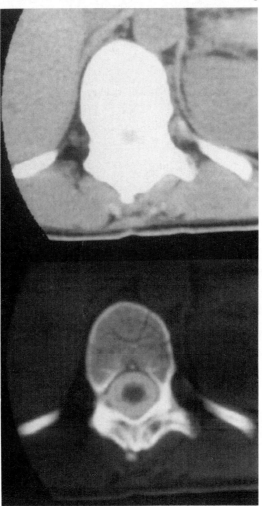

**4-4** Axial CT scan through thoracic spine (T-11) with intrathecal contrast (soft-tissue and bone windows). Section 1 in Fig. 4-3.

# 4/Thoracic Spine, Axial CT

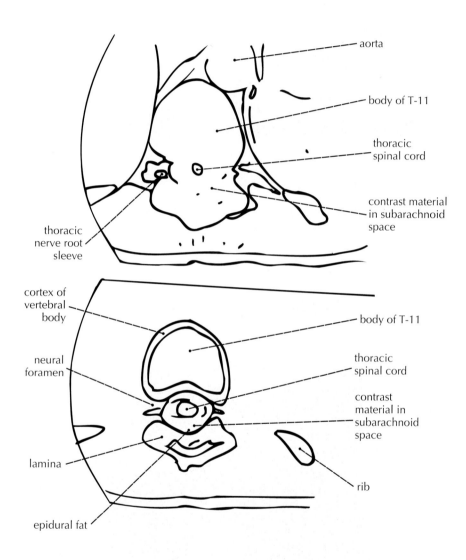

aorta

body of T-11

thoracic
spinal cord

contrast material
in subarachnoid
space

thoracic
nerve root
sleeve

cortex of
vertebral
body

body of T-11

neural
foramen

thoracic
spinal cord

contrast
material in
subarachnoid
space

lamina

rib

epidural fat

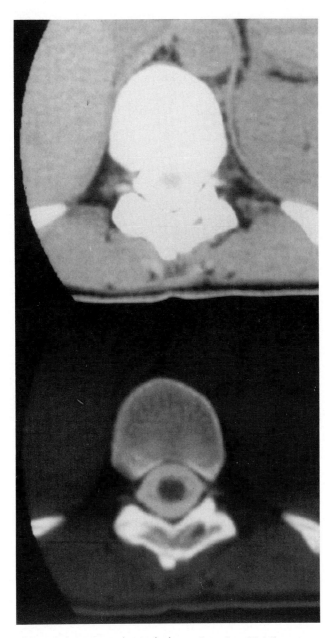

**4-5** Axial CT scan through thoracic spine (T-11) at neural foramen, with intrathecal contrast (soft-tissue and bone windows). Section 2 in Fig. 4-3.

# 4/Thoracic Spine, Sagittal MRI

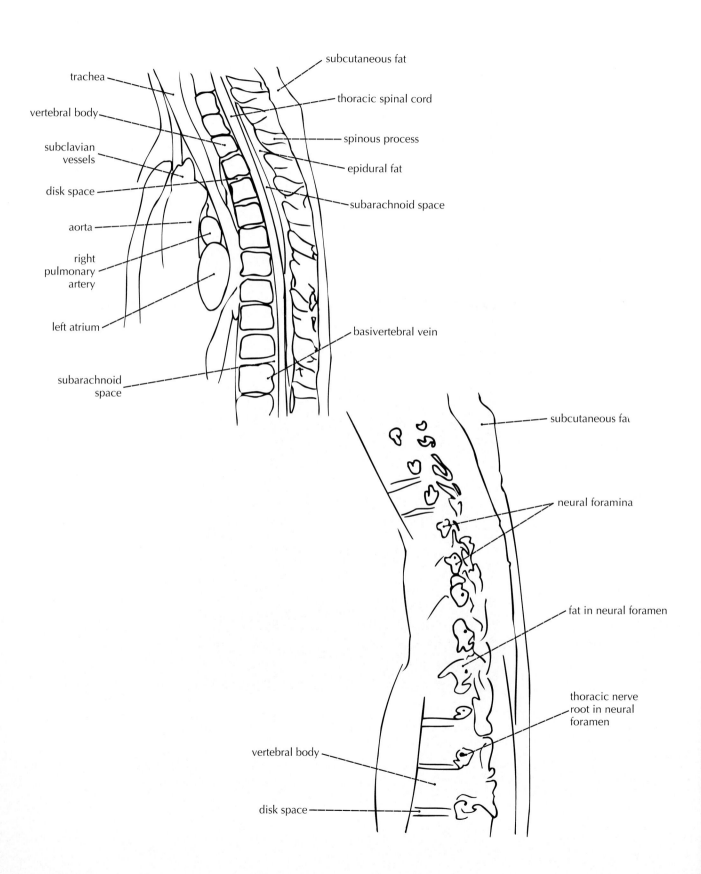

subcutaneous fat

trachea

thoracic spinal cord

vertebral body

spinous process

subclavian
vessels

epidural fat

disk space

subarachnoid space

aorta

right
pulmonary
artery

left atrium

basivertebral vein

subarachnoid
space

subcutaneous fat

neural foramina

fat in neural foramen

thoracic nerve
root in neural
foramen

vertebral body

disk space

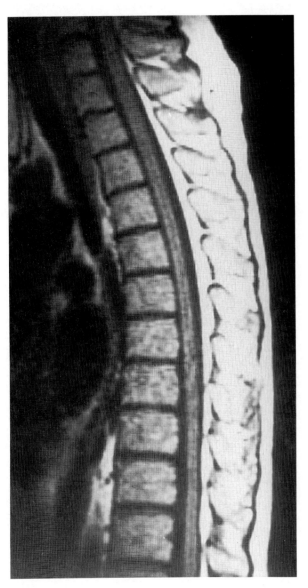

**4-6** Midline sagittal MR scan through thoracic spine (600/20).

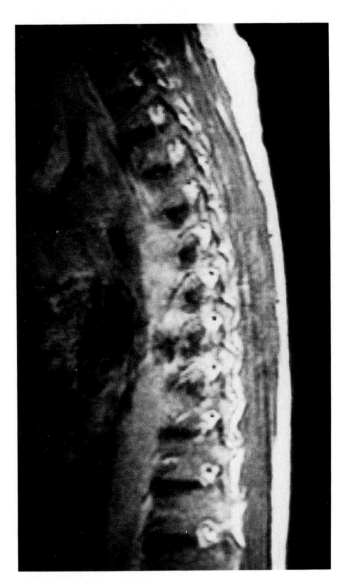

**4-7** Paramidline sagittal MR scan through thoracic spine (2000/30).

# 4/Thoracic Spine, Sagittal MRI

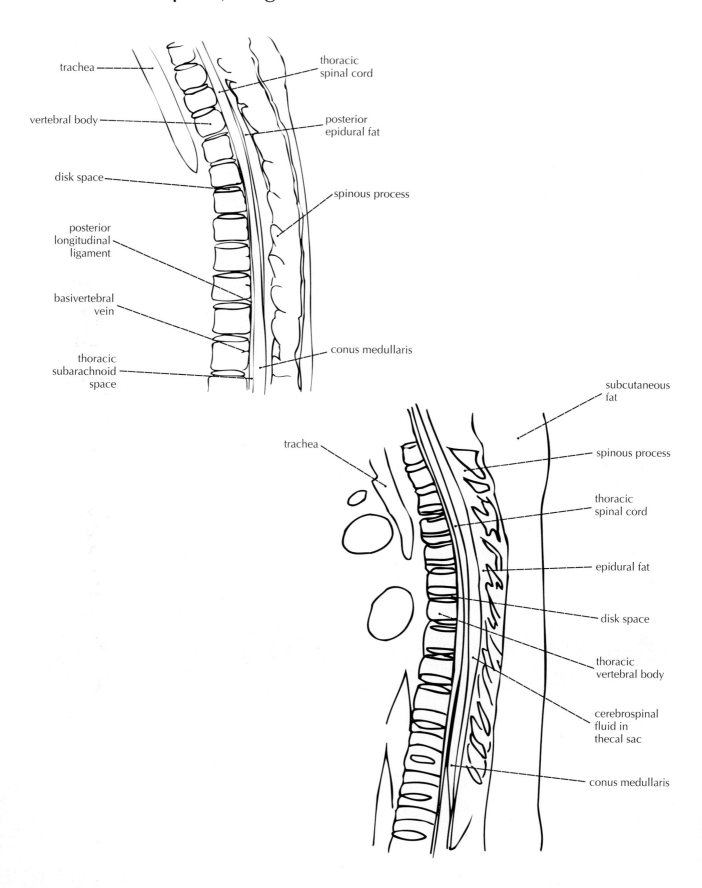

trachea

thoracic spinal cord

vertebral body

posterior epidural fat

disk space

spinous process

posterior longitudinal ligament

basivertebral vein

conus medullaris

thoracic subarachnoid space

trachea

subcutaneous fat

spinous process

thoracic spinal cord

epidural fat

disk space

thoracic vertebral body

cerebrospinal fluid in thecal sac

conus medullaris

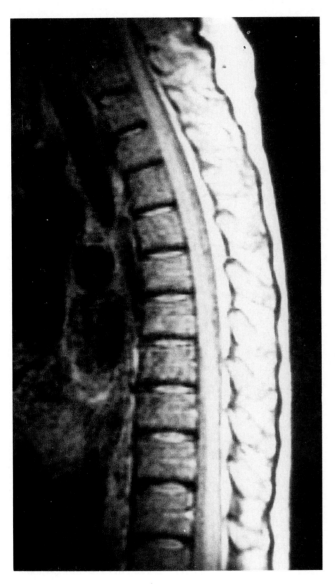

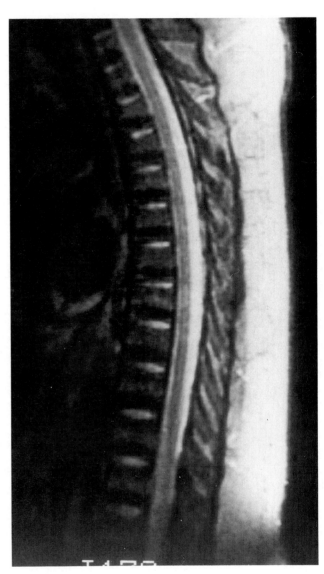

**4-8** Midline sagittal MR scan through thoracic spine (2000/30).

**4-9** Midline sagittal MR scan through thoracic spine (2000/90).

# 4/Thoracic Spine, Sagittal Scout MRI and Coronal MRI

erector spinae muscle

ribs

spinous process

spleen

ligamentum flavum

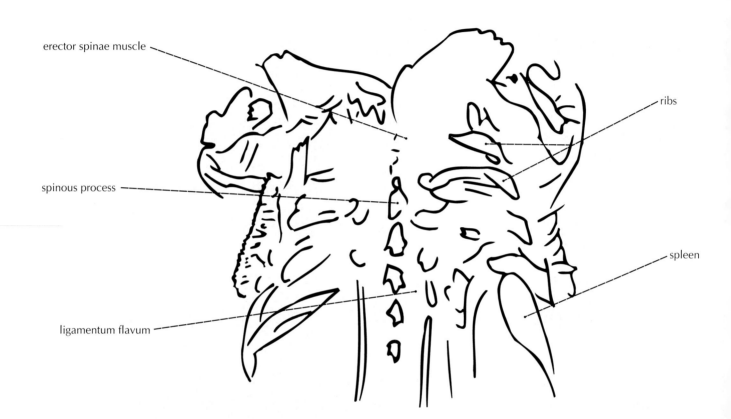

# 4/Thoracic Spine, Sagittal Scout MRI and Coronal MRI

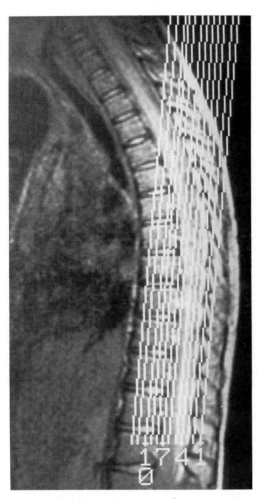

**4-10** Sagittal scout MR scan for orientation of coronal MR scans of thoracic spine. Sections 1, 5, and 9 will be demonstrated (Figs. 4-11–4-13).

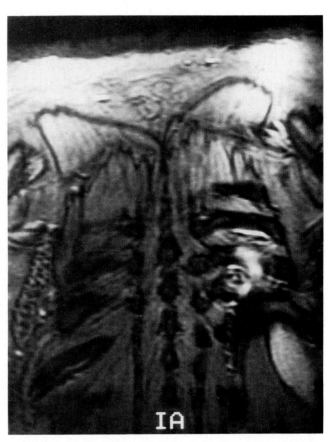

**4-11** Coronal MR scan through posterior thoracic spine (500/18, flip angle 15°) (section 1 in Fig. 4-10).

# 4/Thoracic Spine, Coronal MRI

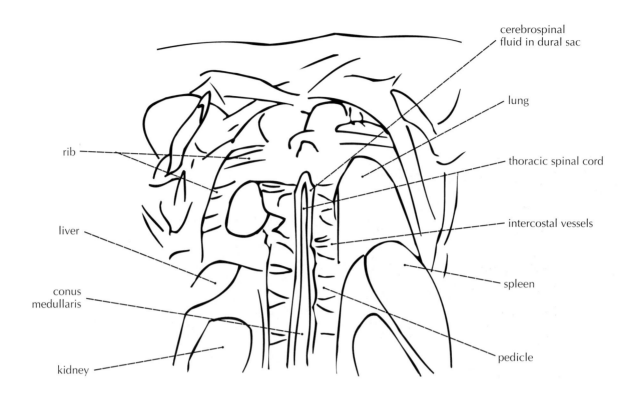

cerebrospinal fluid in dural sac

lung

thoracic spinal cord

intercostal vessels

spleen

pedicle

rib

liver

conus medullaris

kidney

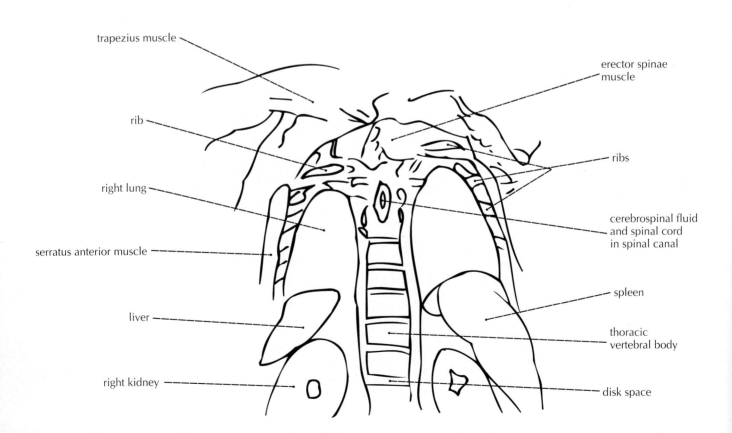

trapezius muscle

erector spinae muscle

rib

ribs

right lung

cerebrospinal fluid and spinal cord in spinal canal

serratus anterior muscle

spleen

liver

thoracic vertebral body

right kidney

disk space

# 4/Thoracic Spine, Coronal MRI

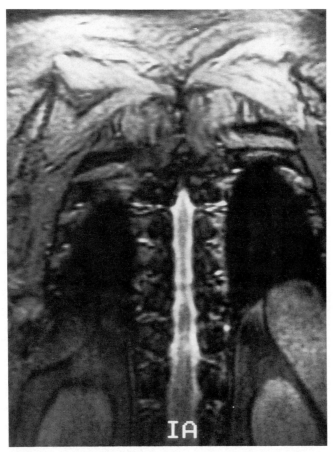

**4-12** Coronal MR scan through thoracic spine (500/18, flip angle 15°) (section 5 in Fig. 4-10).

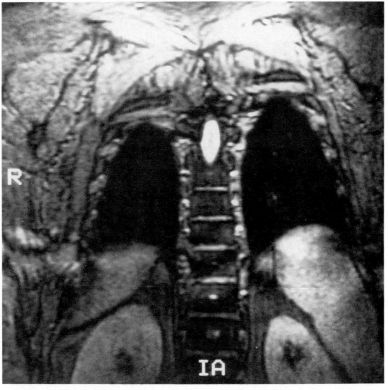

**4-13** Coronal MR scan through thoracic spine (500/18, flip angle 15°) (section 9 in Fig. 4-10).

# 4/Thoracic Spine, Sagittal Scout MRI and Axial MRI

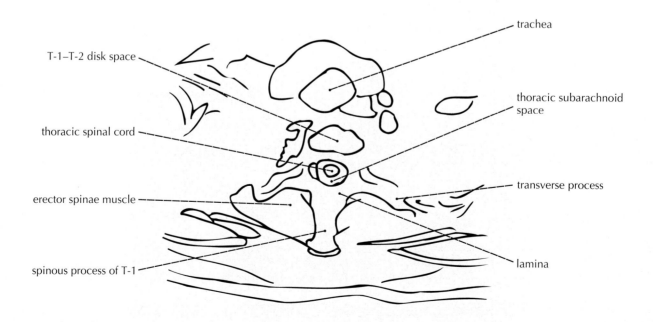

T-1–T-2 disk space

trachea

thoracic subarachnoid space

thoracic spinal cord

erector spinae muscle

transverse process

spinous process of T-1

lamina

# 4/Thoracic Spine, Sagittal Scout MRI and Axial MRI

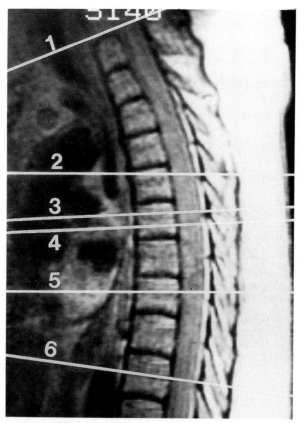

**4-14** Sagittal scout MR for demonstration of the axial images.

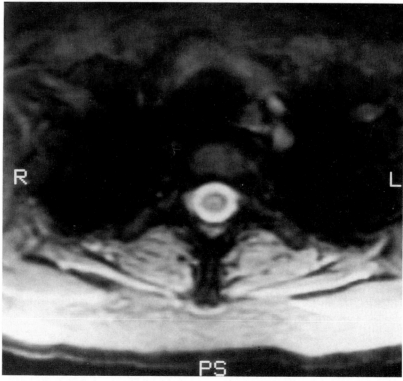

**4-15** Axial MR scan through T-1–T-2 disk space (500/18, flip angle 15°). Section 1 in Fig. 4-14.

# 4/Thoracic Spine, Axial MRI

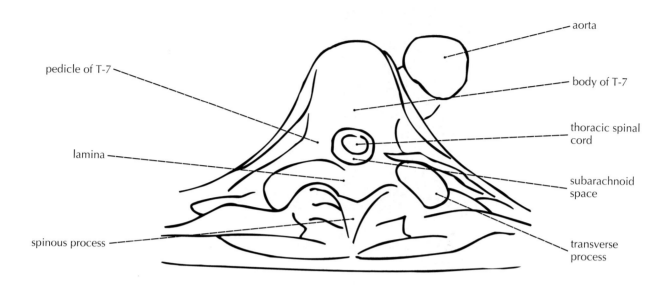

pedicle of T-7

lamina

spinous process

aorta

body of T-7

thoracic spinal cord

subarachnoid space

transverse process

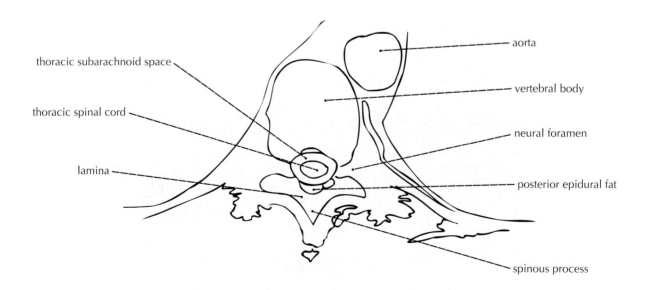

thoracic subarachnoid space

thoracic spinal cord

lamina

aorta

vertebral body

neural foramen

posterior epidural fat

spinous process

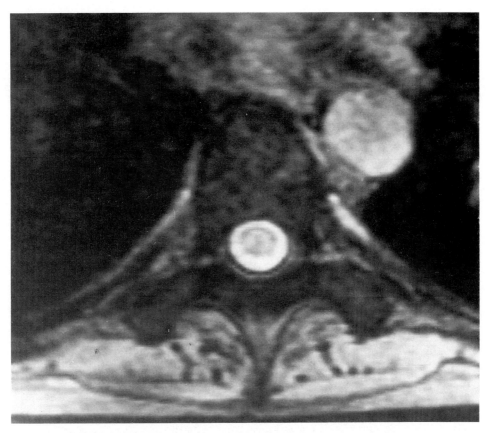

**4-16** Axial MR scan through body of T-7 (500/18, flip angle 15°). Section 3 in Fig. 4-14.

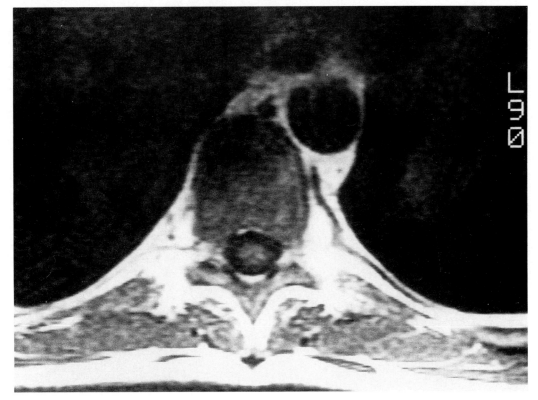

**4-17** Axial MR scan through T-7 (500/20). Section 4 in Fig. 4-14.

# 4/Thoracic Spine, Axial MRI

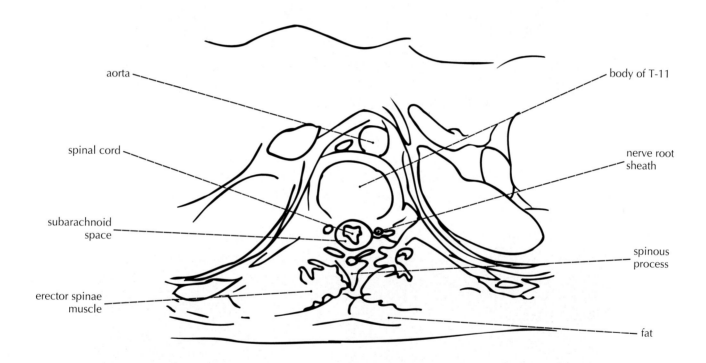

aorta

body of T-11

spinal cord

nerve root
sheath

subarachnoid
space

spinous
process

erector spinae
muscle

fat

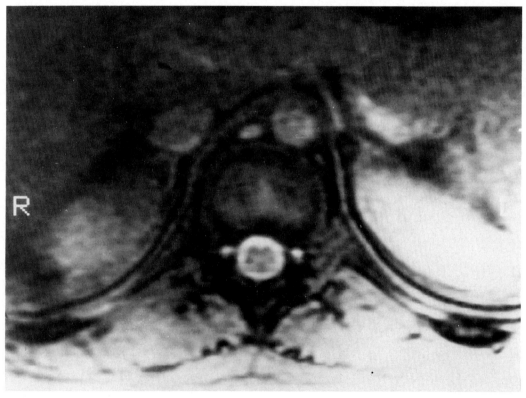

**4-18** Axial MR scan through body of T-11 (500/18, flip angle 15°). Section 6 in Fig. 4-14.

# 4/Thoracic Spine, Myelography

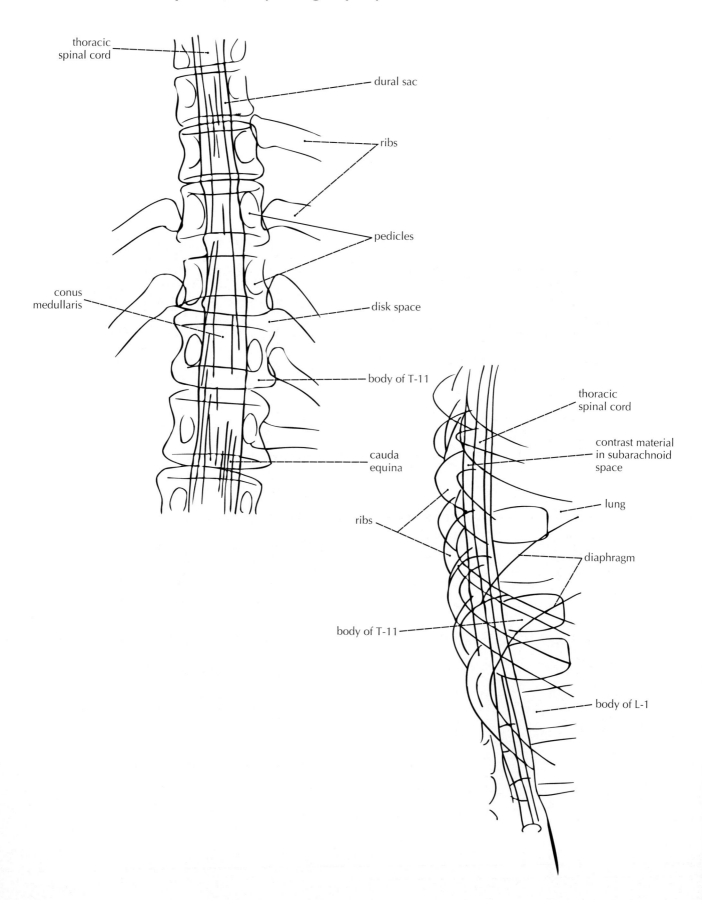

thoracic spinal cord

dural sac

ribs

pedicles

conus medullaris

disk space

body of T-11

cauda equina

ribs

body of T-11

thoracic spinal cord

contrast material in subarachnoid space

lung

diaphragm

body of L-1

# 4/Thoracic Spine, Myelography

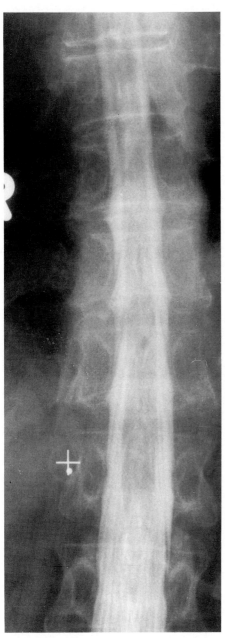

**4-19** Myelogram of thoracic region with conus medullaris, AP view.

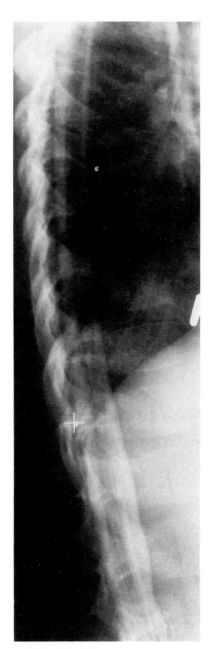

**4-20** Myelogram of lumbothoracic junction, lateral view.

# 5/**Lumbosacral Spine** □ Lumbar Spine, X-Ray

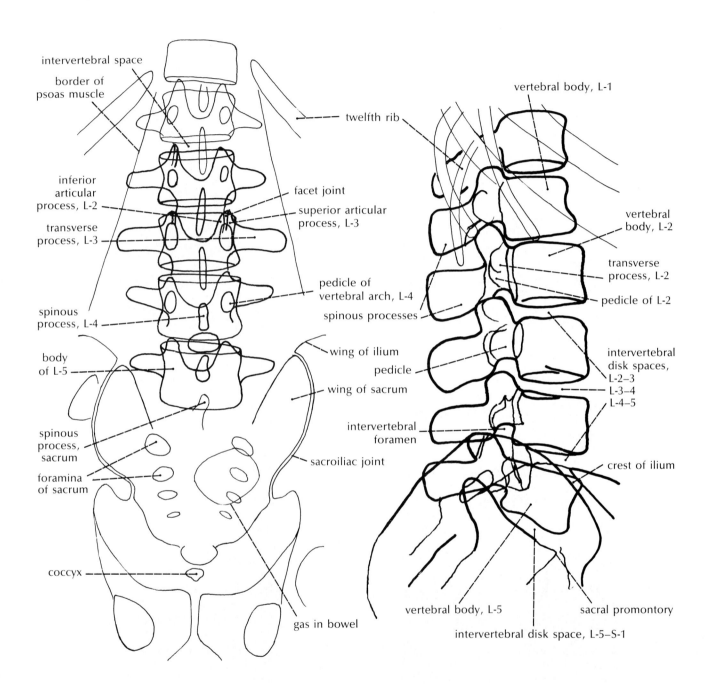

intervertebral space

border of
psoas muscle

twelfth rib

inferior
articular
process, L-2

facet joint

superior articular
process, L-3

transverse
process, L-3

spinous
process, L-4

pedicle of
vertebral arch, L-4

body
of L-5

wing of ilium

spinous processes

wing of sacrum

pedicle

spinous
process,
sacrum

foramina
of sacrum

sacroiliac joint

intervertebral
foramen

coccyx

gas in bowel

vertebral body, L-1

vertebral
body, L-2

transverse
process, L-2

pedicle of L-2

intervertebral
disk spaces,
L-2–3
L-3–4
L-4–5

crest of ilium

vertebral body, L-5

sacral promontory

intervertebral disk space, L-5–S-1

# 5/Lumbar Spine, X-Ray

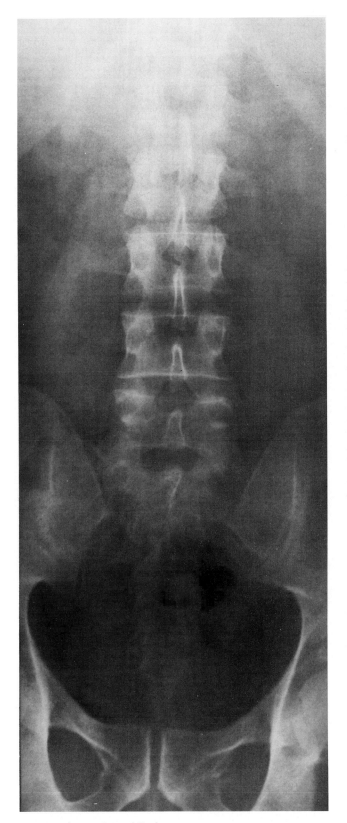

**5-1** Lumbar spine, AP view.

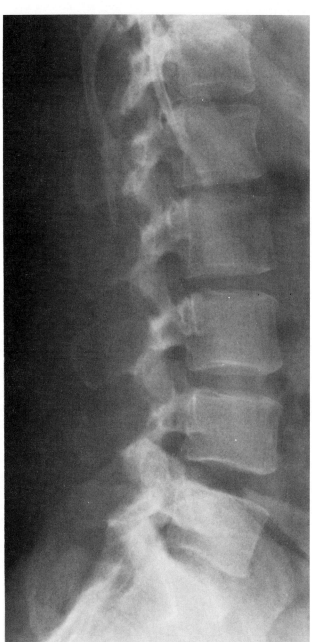

**5-2** Lumbar spine, lateral view.

# 5/Lumbar Spine and Sacroiliac Joint, X-Ray

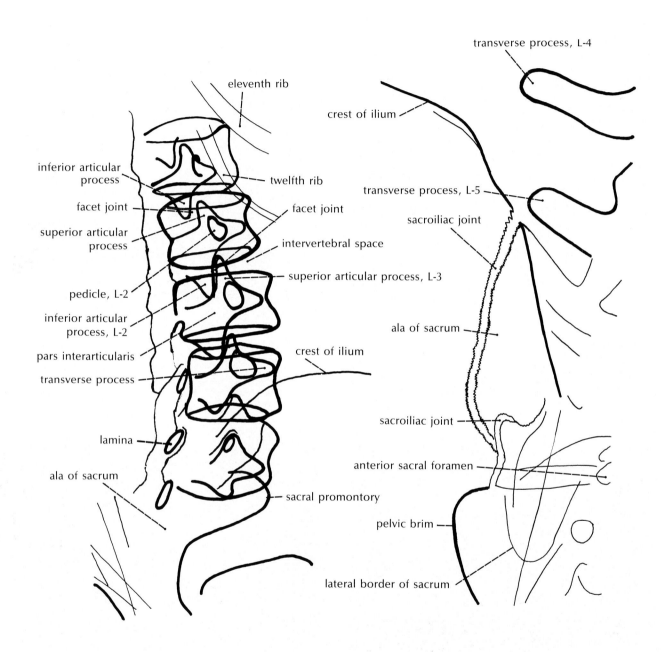

transverse process, L-4

crest of ilium

eleventh rib

inferior articular process

twelfth rib

facet joint

facet joint

transverse process, L-5

sacroiliac joint

superior articular process

intervertebral space

superior articular process, L-3

pedicle, L-2

ala of sacrum

inferior articular process, L-2

pars interarticularis

transverse process

crest of ilium

sacroiliac joint

anterior sacral foramen

lamina

pelvic brim

ala of sacrum

sacral promontory

lateral border of sacrum

# 5/Lumbar Spine and Sacroiliac Joint, X-Ray

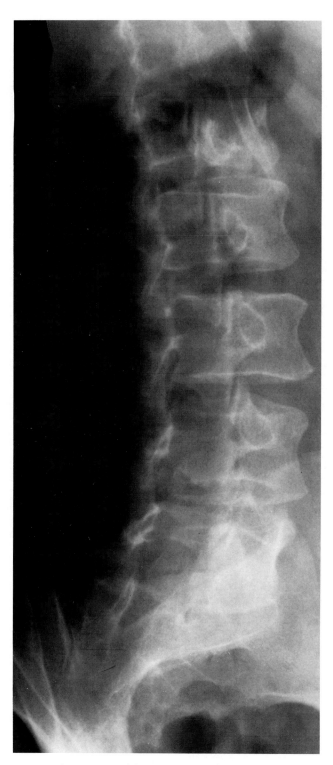

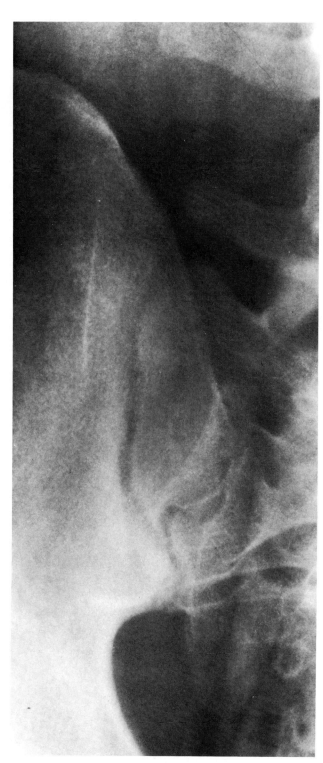

5-3 Lumbar spine, oblique view (reduced in size compared with Fig. 5-4).

5-4 Sacroiliac joint, oblique view.

# 5/Sacrum and Coccyx, X-Ray

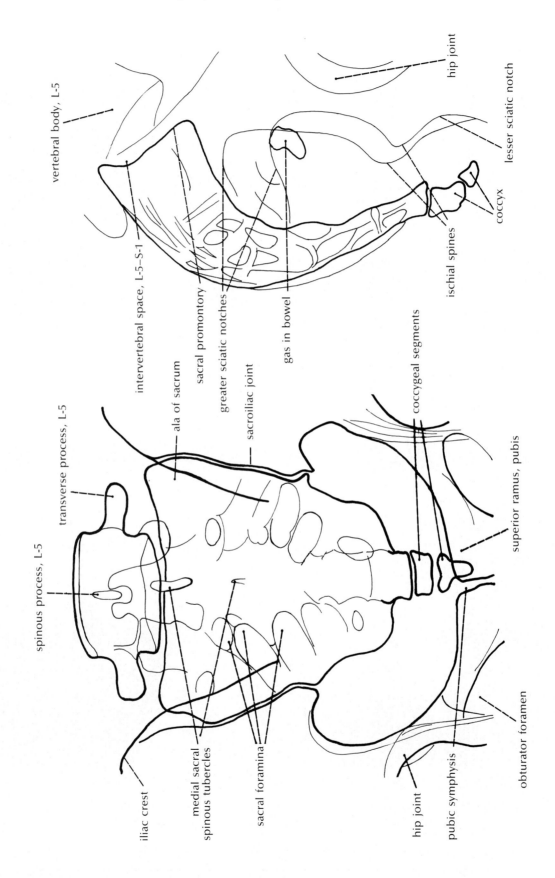

vertebral body, L-5

hip joint

lesser sciatic notch

coccyx

ischial spines

intervertebral space, L-5–S-1

ala of sacrum

sacral promontory

greater sciatic notches

sacroiliac joint

gas in bowel

coccygeal segments

transverse process, L-5

superior ramus, pubis

spinous process, L-5

iliac crest

medial sacral spinous tubercles

sacral foramina

hip joint

pubic symphysis

obturator foramen

# 5/Sacrum and Coccyx, X-Ray

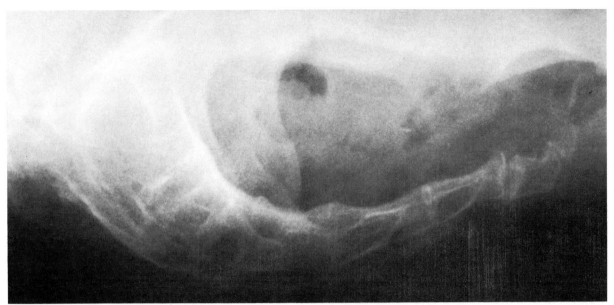

5-6 Sacrum and coccyx, lateral view.

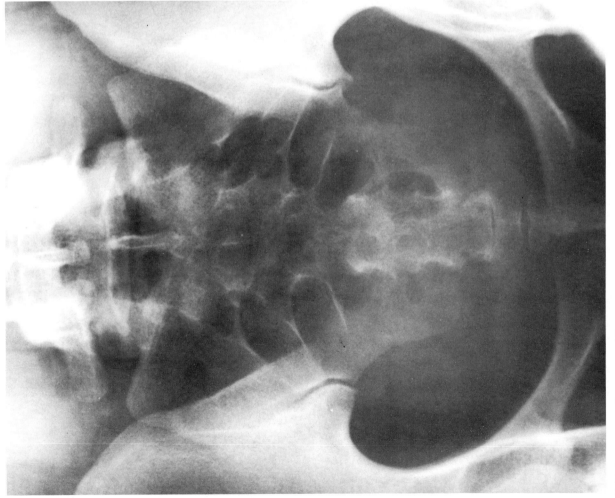

5-5 Sacrum and coccyx, AP view.

# 5/Lumbosacral Spine, Sagittal Scout CT and Axial CT

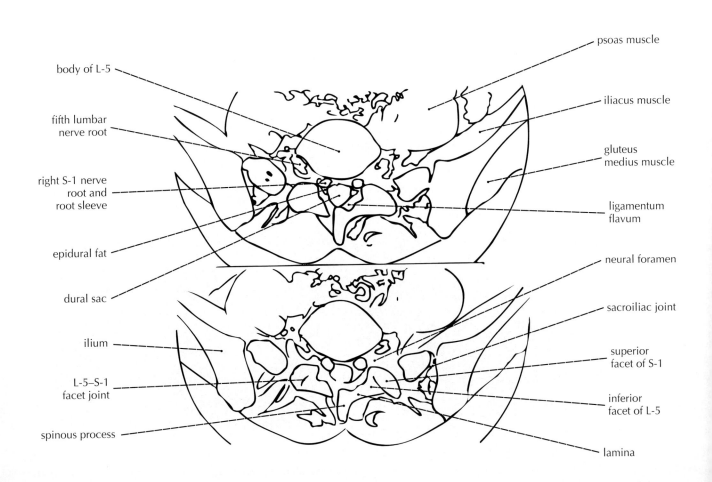

body of L-5

fifth lumbar
nerve root

right S-1 nerve
root and
root sleeve

epidural fat

dural sac

ilium

L-5–S-1
facet joint

spinous process

psoas muscle

iliacus muscle

gluteus
medius muscle

ligamentum
flavum

neural foramen

sacroiliac joint

superior
facet of S-1

inferior
facet of L-5

lamina

# 5/Lumbosacral Spine, Sagittal Scout CT and Axial CT

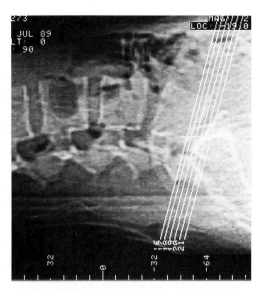

**5-7** Sagittal scout CT scan for orientation of axial CT scans at L-5–S-1 disk space. Section 16 (the uppermost section) will be demonstrated in Fig. 5-8.

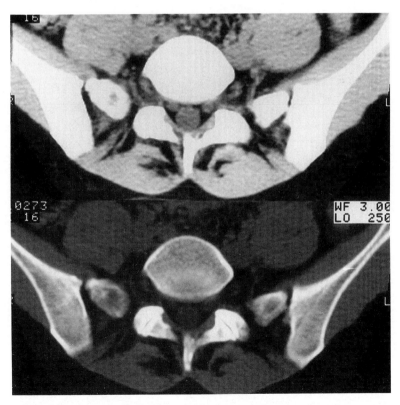

**5-8** Axial CT scan through L-5–S-1 level (soft-tissue and bone windows) (section 16 in Fig. 5-7).

# 5/Lumbosacral Spine, Sagittal Scout CT and Axial CT

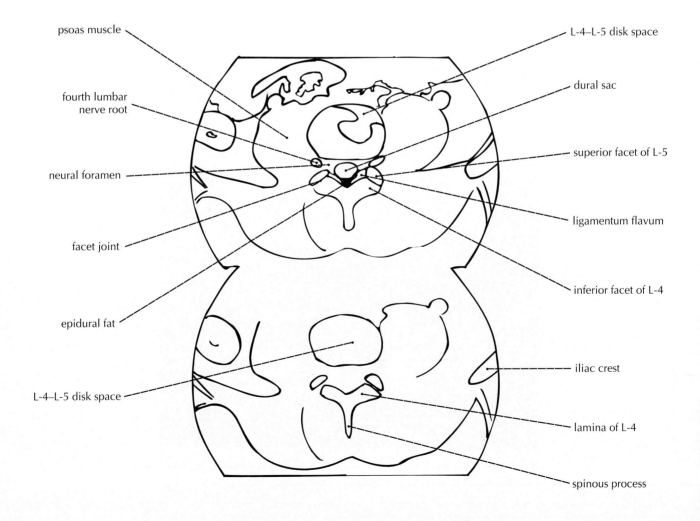

psoas muscle

L-4–L-5 disk space

fourth lumbar
nerve root

dural sac

superior facet of L-5

neural foramen

ligamentum flavum

facet joint

inferior facet of L-4

epidural fat

iliac crest

L-4–L-5 disk space

lamina of L-4

spinous process

# 5/Lumbosacral Spine, Sagittal Scout CT and Axial CT

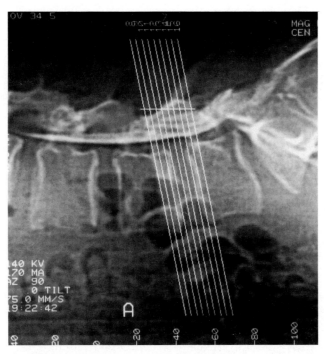

**5-9** Sagittal scout CT scan with intrathecal contrast for orientation of axial CT scans through L-4 and through L-4–L-5 disk space. Sections 11, 9 and 12 will be demonstrated in Figs. 5-10, 5-11 and 5-12.

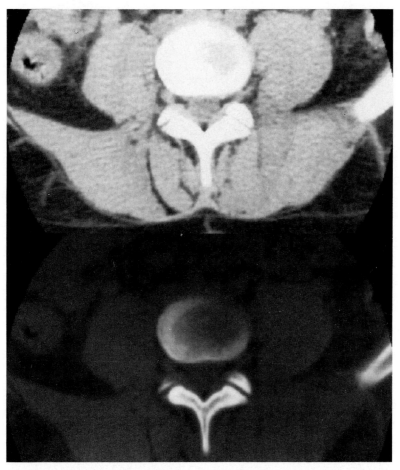

**5-10** Axial CT scan through L-4–L-5 disk space (soft-tissue and bone windows). Section 11 in scout 5-10. A noncontrast scan.

# 5/Lumbosacral Spine, Axial CT

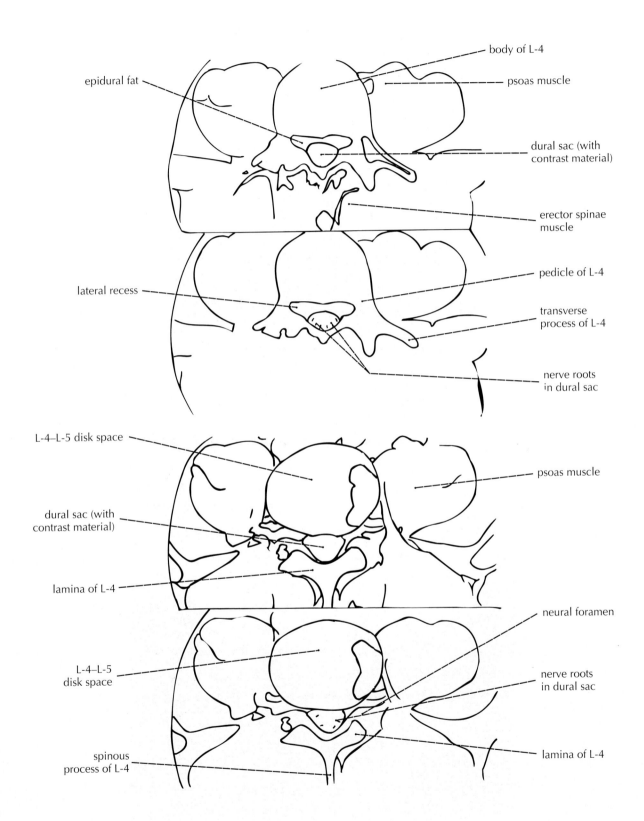

body of L-4

psoas muscle

epidural fat

dural sac (with contrast material)

erector spinae muscle

pedicle of L-4

lateral recess

transverse process of L-4

nerve roots in dural sac

L-4–L-5 disk space

psoas muscle

dural sac (with contrast material)

lamina of L-4

neural foramen

L-4–L-5 disk space

nerve roots in dural sac

spinous process of L-4

lamina of L-4

# 5/Lumbosacral Spine, Axial CT

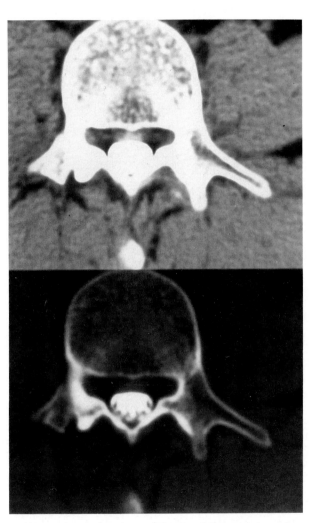

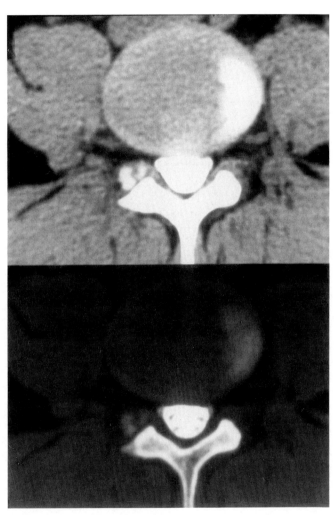

**5-11** Axial CT scan through body of L-4 with intrathecal contrast (soft-tissue and bone windows) (section 9 in Fig. 5-9).

**5-12** Axial CT scan through L-4–L-5 disk space with intrathecal contrast (soft-tissue and bone windows) (section 12 in Fig. 5-9).

# 5/Lumbosacral Spine, Sagittal Scout CT and Axial CT

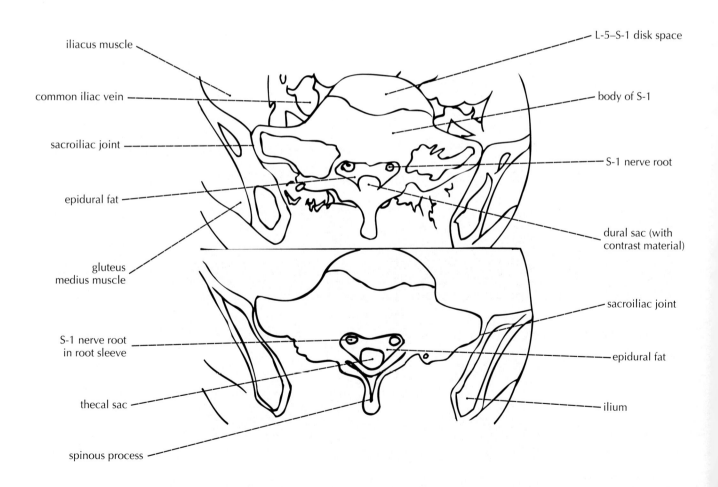

iliacus muscle

common iliac vein

sacroiliac joint

epidural fat

gluteus
medius muscle

S-1 nerve root
in root sleeve

thecal sac

spinous process

L-5–S-1 disk space

body of S-1

S-1 nerve root

dural sac (with
contrast material)

sacroiliac joint

epidural fat

ilium

# 5/Lumbosacral Spine, Sagittal Scout CT and Axial CT

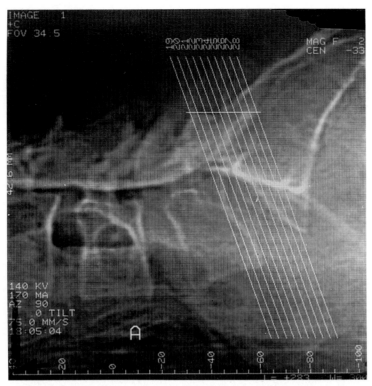

**5-13** Sagittal scout CT scan with intrathecal contrast through L-5–S-1 disk space for orientation of axial CT scans. Section 25 will be demonstrated in Fig. 5-14.

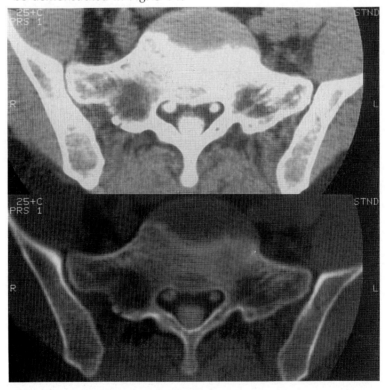

**5-14** Axial CT scan through body of S-1 with intrathecal contrast (soft-tissue and bone windows) (section 25 in Fig. 5-13).

# 5/Lumbosacral Spine, MRI

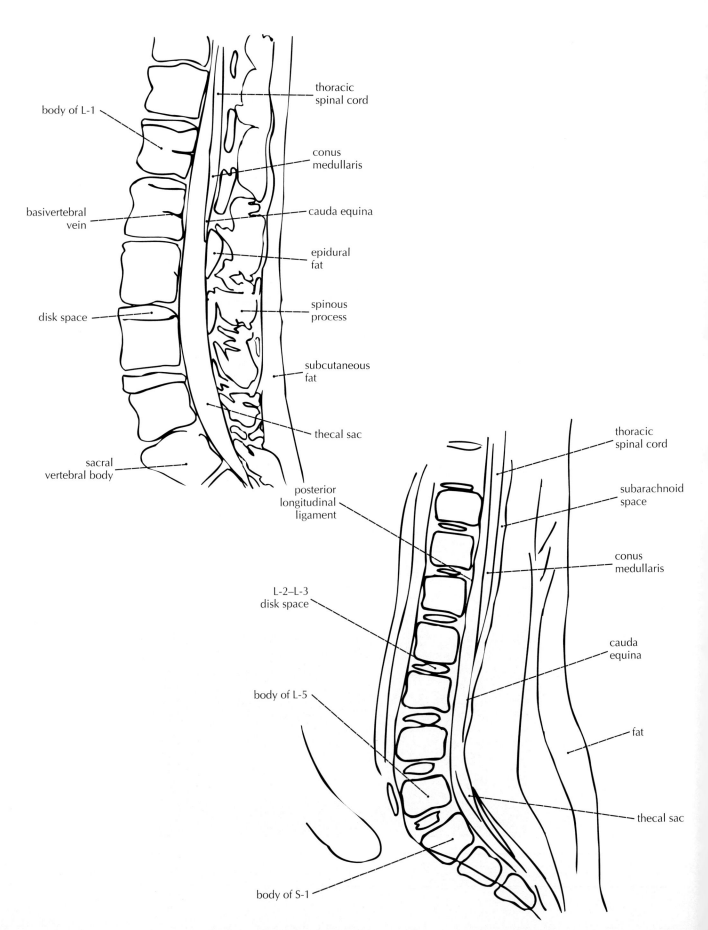

body of L-1

basivertebral
vein

disk space

sacral
vertebral body

thoracic
spinal cord

conus
medullaris

cauda equina

epidural
fat

spinous
process

subcutaneous
fat

thecal sac

posterior
longitudinal
ligament

L-2–L-3
disk space

body of L-5

body of S-1

thoracic
spinal cord

subarachnoid
space

conus
medullaris

cauda
equina

fat

thecal sac

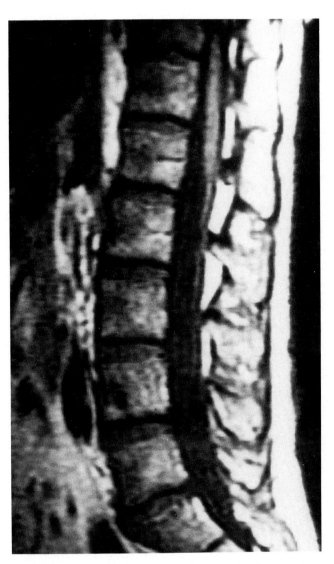

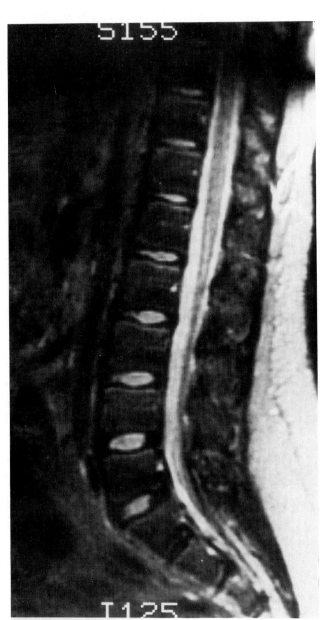

**5-15** Midline sagittal MR scan through lumbosacral region (600/20).

**5-16** Midline sagittal MR scan through lumbar region (2000/90).

# 5/Lumbosacral Spine, MRI

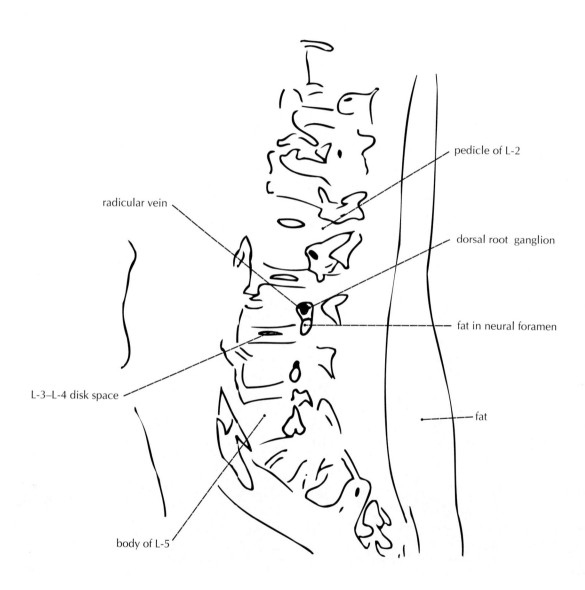

radicular vein

pedicle of L-2

dorsal root ganglion

fat in neural foramen

L-3–L-4 disk space

fat

body of L-5

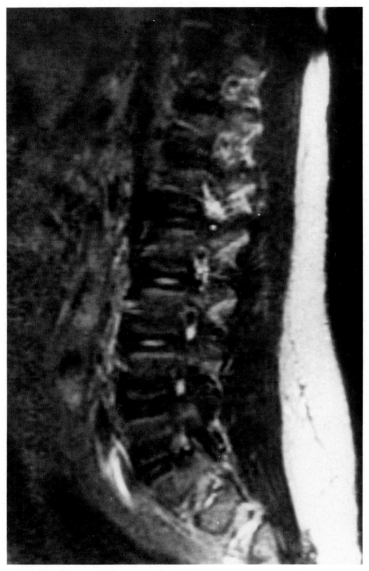

**5-17** Paramidline sagittal MR scan through lumbar region (2000/90).

# 5/Lumbosacral Spine, Sagittal Scout MRI and Coronal MRI

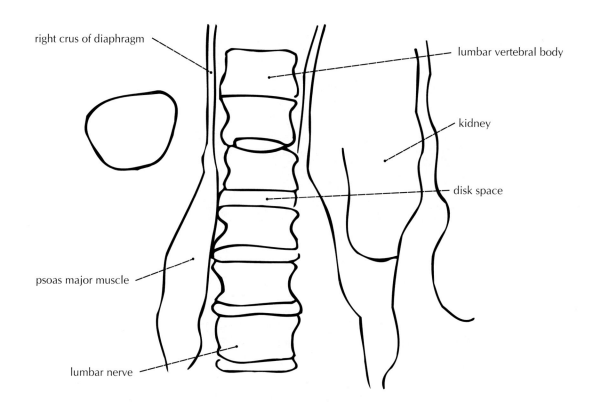

right crus of diaphragm

lumbar vertebral body

kidney

disk space

psoas major muscle

lumbar nerve

# 5/Lumbosacral Spine, Sagittal Scout MRI and Coronal MRI

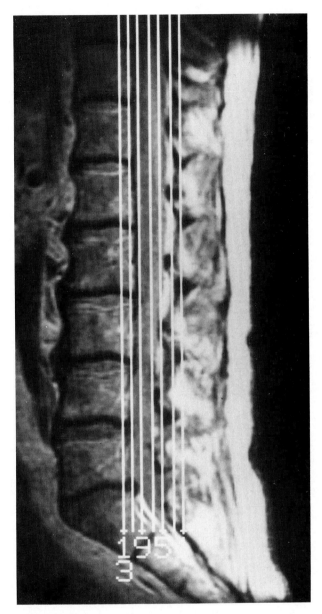

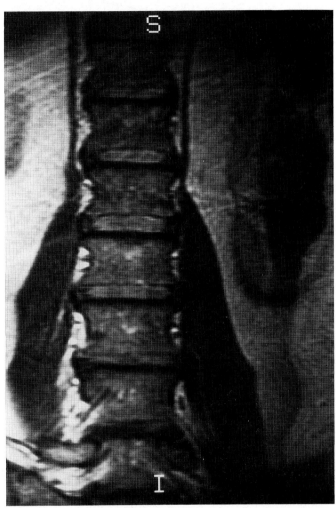

**5-18** Sagittal scout MR scan used for demonstration of selected coronal images. Sections 13, 7 and 1 will be shown.

**5-19** Coronal MR scan through lumbar spinal canal (2000/30). Section 13 in Fig. 5-18.

# 5/Lumbosacral Spine, Coronal MRI

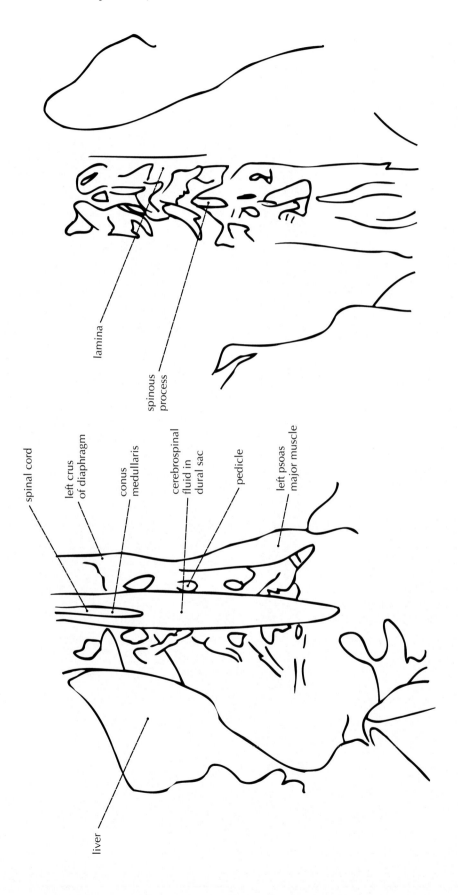

lamina

spinous process

spinal cord

left crus of diaphragm

conus medullaris

cerebrospinal fluid in dural sac

pedicle

left psoas major muscle

liver

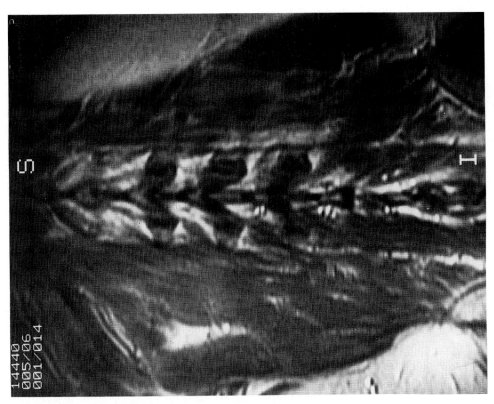

**5-21** Coronal MR scan through lumbar spinal canal (2000/30). Section 1 in Fig. 5-18.

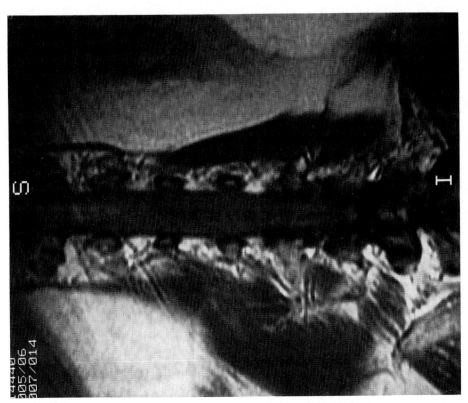

**5-20** Coronal MR scan through lumbar spinal canal (2000/30). Section 7 in Fig. 5-18.

# 5/Lumbosacral Spine, Sagittal Scout MRI and Axial MRI

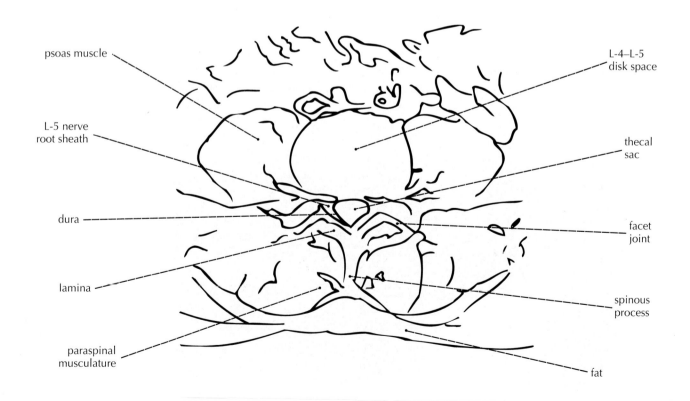

psoas muscle

L-5 nerve
root sheath

dura

lamina

paraspinal
musculature

L-4–L-5
disk space

thecal
sac

facet
joint

spinous
process

fat

# 5/Lumbosacral Spine, Sagittal Scout MRI and Axial MRI

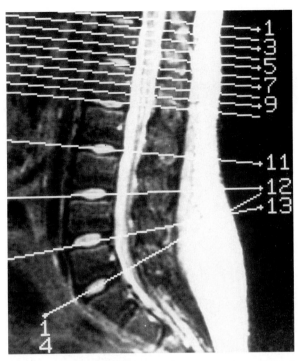

**5-22** Sagittal scout MR scan for orientation of axial MR scans of the lumbosacral spine.

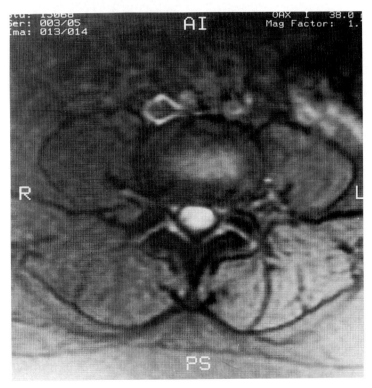

**5-23** Axial MR scan through L-4–L-5 disk space (500/18, flip angle 15°) (section 13 in Fig. 5-22).

# 5/Lumbosacral Spine, Axial MRI

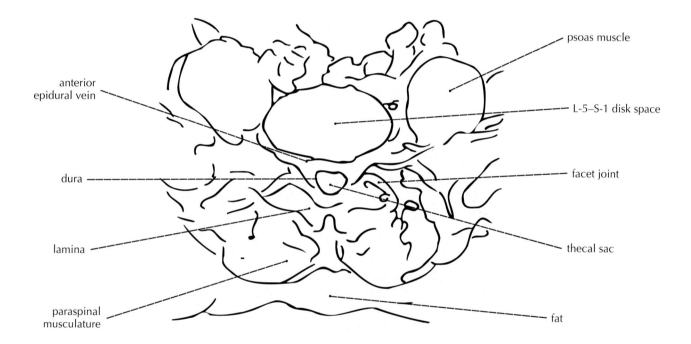

anterior epidural vein

psoas muscle

L-5–S-1 disk space

dura

facet joint

lamina

thecal sac

paraspinal musculature

fat

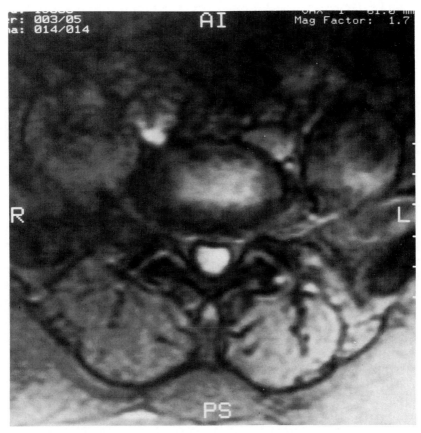

**5-24** Axial MR scan through L-5—S-1 disk space (500/18, flip angle 15°) (section 14 in Fig. 5-22).

# 5/Thoracolumbar Spine, Myelography

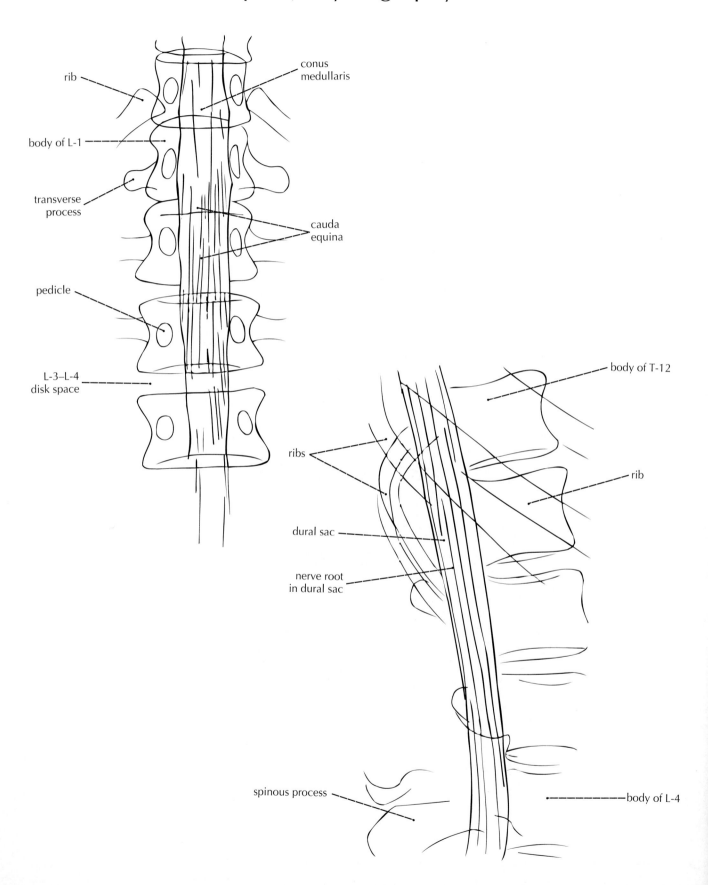

# 5/Thoracolumbar Spine, Myelography

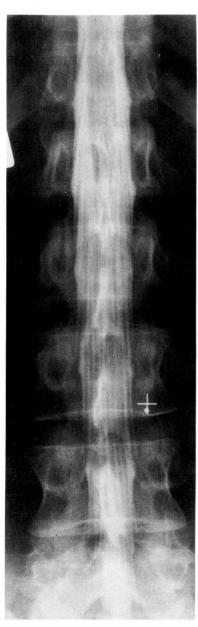

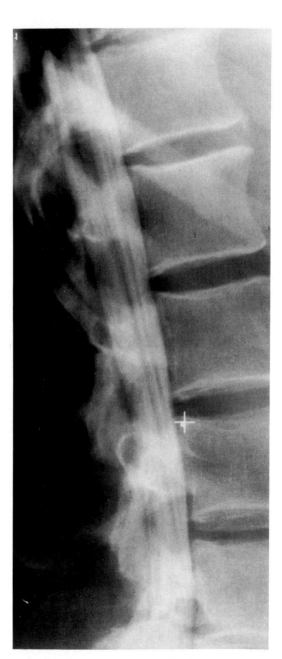

**5-25** Myelogram of thoracolumbar region, AP view.

**5-26** Myelogram of thoracolumbar region, lateral view.

# 5/Lumbosacral Spine, Myelography

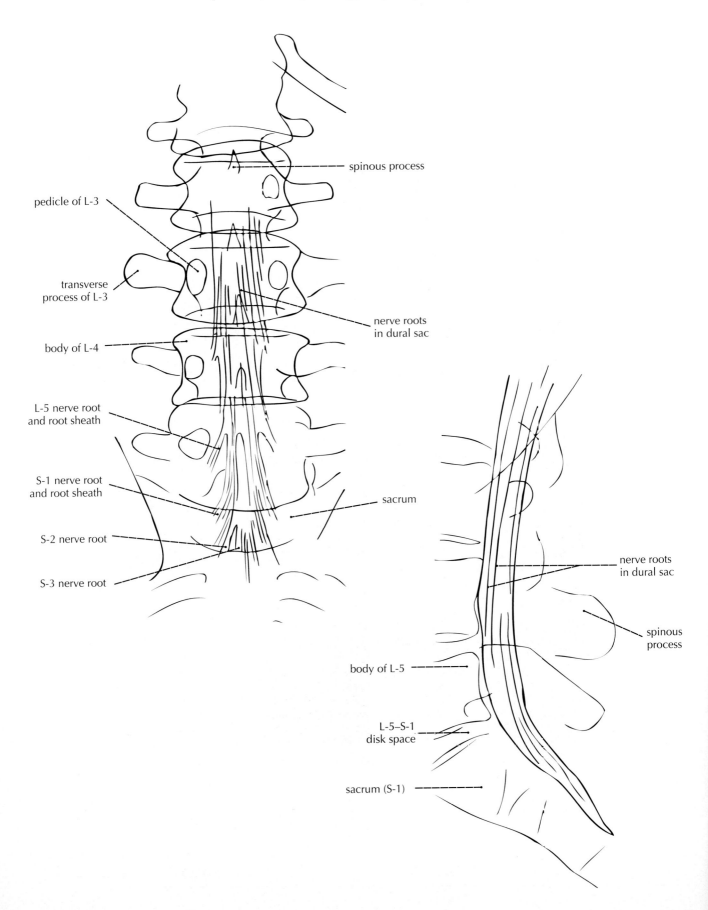

spinous process

pedicle of L-3

transverse process of L-3

nerve roots in dural sac

body of L-4

L-5 nerve root and root sheath

S-1 nerve root and root sheath

sacrum

S-2 nerve root

S-3 nerve root

nerve roots in dural sac

spinous process

body of L-5

L-5–S-1 disk space

sacrum (S-1)

# 5/Lumbosacral Spine, Myelography

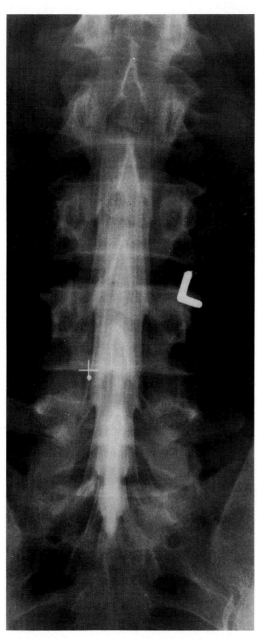

**5-27** Myelogram of lumbosacral region, AP view.

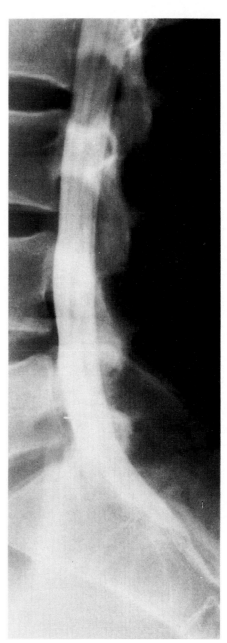

**5-28** Myelogram of lumbosacral region, lateral view.

# 5/Lumbosacral Spine, Myelography

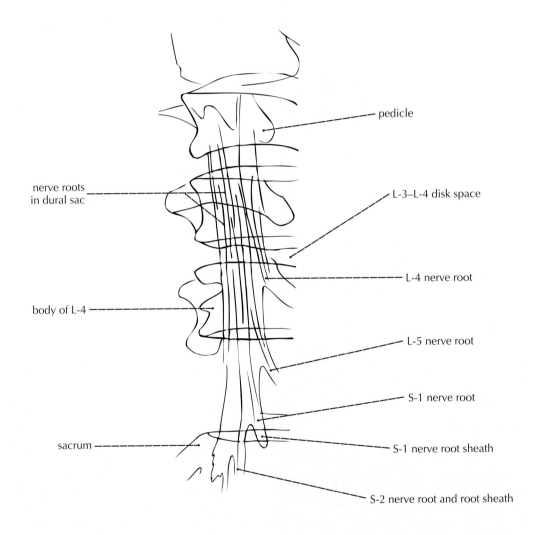

pedicle

nerve roots
in dural sac

L-3–L-4 disk space

L-4 nerve root

body of L-4

L-5 nerve root

S-1 nerve root

sacrum

S-1 nerve root sheath

S-2 nerve root and root sheath

# 5/Lumbosacral Spine, Myelography

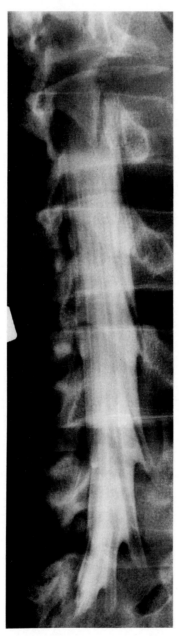

**5-29** Myelogram of lumbosacral region, oblique view.